INDIA: ECONOMIC, POLITICAL AND SOCIAL ISSUES

# WEST BENGAL

# ECONOMIC, POLITICAL AND SOCIAL ISSUES

# INDIA: ECONOMIC, POLITICAL AND SOCIAL ISSUES

Additional books and e-books in this series can be found on Nova's website under the Series tab.

INDIA: ECONOMIC, POLITICAL AND SOCIAL ISSUES

# WEST BENGAL

## ECONOMIC, POLITICAL AND SOCIAL ISSUES

RHIANU BOWELL
EDITOR

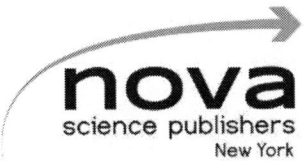

nova science publishers
New York

Copyright © 2021 by Nova Science Publishers, Inc.

**All rights reserved.** No part of this book may be reproduced, stored in a retrieval system or transmitted in any form or by any means: electronic, electrostatic, magnetic, tape, mechanical photocopying, recording or otherwise without the written permission of the Publisher.

We have partnered with Copyright Clearance Center to make it easy for you to obtain permissions to reuse content from this publication. Simply navigate to this publication's page on Nova's website and locate the "Get Permission" button below the title description. This button is linked directly to the title's permission page on copyright.com. Alternatively, you can visit copyright.com and search by title, ISBN, or ISSN.

For further questions about using the service on copyright.com, please contact:
Copyright Clearance Center
Phone: +1-(978) 750-8400        Fax: +1-(978) 750-4470        E-mail: info@copyright.com.

### NOTICE TO THE READER

The Publisher has taken reasonable care in the preparation of this book, but makes no expressed or implied warranty of any kind and assumes no responsibility for any errors or omissions. No liability is assumed for incidental or consequential damages in connection with or arising out of information contained in this book. The Publisher shall not be liable for any special, consequential, or exemplary damages resulting, in whole or in part, from the readers' use of, or reliance upon, this material. Any parts of this book based on government reports are so indicated and copyright is claimed for those parts to the extent applicable to compilations of such works.

Independent verification should be sought for any data, advice or recommendations contained in this book. In addition, no responsibility is assumed by the Publisher for any injury and/or damage to persons or property arising from any methods, products, instructions, ideas or otherwise contained in this publication.

This publication is designed to provide accurate and authoritative information with regard to the subject matter covered herein. It is sold with the clear understanding that the Publisher is not engaged in rendering legal or any other professional services. If legal or any other expert assistance is required, the services of a competent person should be sought. FROM A DECLARATION OF PARTICIPANTS JOINTLY ADOPTED BY A COMMITTEE OF THE AMERICAN BAR ASSOCIATION AND A COMMITTEE OF PUBLISHERS.

Additional color graphics may be available in the e-book version of this book.

## Library of Congress Cataloging-in-Publication Data

ISBN: 978-1-53619-237-7

*Published by Nova Science Publishers, Inc. † New York*

# CONTENTS

| | | |
|---|---|---|
| **Preface** | | vii |
| **Chapter 1** | Lifestyle Induced Addictive Habits: A Socio-Physiological Issue of Kolkata, West Bengal<br>*Gouriprosad Datta, Anurupa Sen, Moumita Das and Subhashree Basu* | 1 |
| **Chapter 2** | MGNREGA and Women Empowerment: Socio-Economic Implications<br>*Arindam Chakraborty* | 63 |
| **Chapter 3** | Age Trends in Anthropometric Characteristics and Nutritional Status among Adult Mahali Females of Bankura District, West Bengal, India<br>*Kaushik Bose, Shilpita Bhandar, Mihir Ghosh, Binoy Kumar Kuiti, Soma Pal and Swarup Pratihar* | 81 |
| **Index** | | 99 |

# PREFACE

Globally, industrialization and urbanization are leading to improvement in society's economic condition which is often accompanied by lifestyle changes including physical inactivity, unhealthy diet and harmful use of tobacco and alcohol. These altered lifestyles bring about non-communicable diseases (NCDs) like obesity, hypertension (HTN) and diabetes mellitus (DM). The risk factors of the lifestyle induced NCDs are measurable and largely modifiable. So, continuous surveillance on the levels and patterns of risk factors is of fundamental importance to control NCDs. Chapter 1 focuses on this and conducted a study on 1216 male individuals of different socio-economic status residing at Kolkata, West Bengal.

The Mahatma Gandhi National Rural Employment Guarantee Act (MGNREGA) was initiated in India in 2006 with a view to creating more wage employment in rural areas thereby ameliorating rural poverty. But after the completion of more than a decade, the effects and roles of the scheme are found to be manifolds. Particularly, if we consider the impact of women. Chapter 2 looks at how the role of women have changed, especially in the family, and how that impacts society.

In chapter 3, the authors performed a study to assess age trends in anthropometric measures and nutritional status among adult Mahali females. It was a community-based cross-sectional study, carried out in selected four villages of Bankura district, West Bengal, India.

Chapter 1 - Globally, industrialization and urbanization are leading to improvement in society's economic condition which is often accompanied by lifestyle changes including physical inactivity, unhealthy diet and harmful use of tobacco and alcohol. These altered lifestyles bring about non-communicable diseases (NCDs) like obesity, hypertension (HTN) and diabetes mellitus (DM). The risk factors of the lifestyle induced NCDs are measurable and largely modifiable. So, continuous surveillance on the levels and patterns of risk factors is of fundamental importance to control NCDs. The study was conducted on 1216 male individuals of different socio-economic status residing at Kolkata, West Bengal, with age ranged 20–60 years. WHO STEP-wise tool was used for face-to-face interviews and a suitably modified WHO-NCD risk factor questionnaire was employed. Personal information regarding physical activity, smoking, smokeless tobacco (SLT) and alcohol consumption along with the personal and family history of HTN and DM were recorded. All the physiological and anthropometric variables were measured using standard procedures. The cutoff values provided by WHO, JNC-VII and ADA were used to classify obesity, HTN and DM, respectively. Different body composition analysis and somatotyping were also done. All statistical computations were performed with SPSS 20.0. For all analyses, $p < 0.05$ were considered as statistically significant. Smoking, SLT use, alcohol consumption and physical inactivity were observed among 39.1%, 26.7%, 30% and 72.9% people, respectively. Current smokers had increased heart rate (HR), systolic blood pressure (SBP), diastolic blood pressure (DBP) and random blood sugar (RBS) values whereas body mass index (BMI) and waist circumference (WC) decreased with increase in number of cigarettes smoked/day. The increase in drinking quantity significantly increased SBP, DBP, WC and waist-hip ratio (WHR) values. RBS was the highest among light drinkers whereas BMI was the highest among heavy drinkers. Highest DBP and SBP value were observed in 'Alcoholic' and 'Smoker-Alcoholic' group, respectively. 'Smoker-Alcoholic' group had highest mean value of RBS and lowest value was noticed in 'Alcoholic' group. BMI, WC and

WHR were also significantly higher in 'Alcoholic' group. All skinfold (SKF) thicknesses, muscle girths, percent body fat (%BF), fat mass (FM), percent muscle mass (%MM), muscle mass (MM), endomorphy and mesomorphy rating decreased with increase in cigarettes smoked/day while ectomorphy rating showed a reverse trend. All the muscle girths, bone widths, skeletal mass (SM), MM, abdominal SKF, FM and lean body mass (LBM) values showed a linear increasing pattern with increase in alcohol consumption whereas subscapular and mid-thigh SKFs showed a decreasing trend. Moreover, all the alcoholics were mesomorphic endomorph. Highest mean values of FM and LBM were found in the 'Alcoholic' group. They also had higher MM, percent skeletal mass (%SM) and SM. Additionally, 'Alcoholics were less ectomorphic, 'Smokers were less mesomorphic and 'Smoker-alcoholics were less endomorphic. The changed lifestyle demonstrated severe impact on prevalence of NCDs and they also significantly changed the anthropometric and body composition parameters as well as the somatotype ratings. Avoidance to addiction and changes in lifestyle could be an important intervention in preventing/delaying the ongoing upswing in prevalence of NCDs and their associated risk factors.

Chapter 2 - The Mahatma Gandhi National Rural Employment Guarantee Act (MGNREGA) was initiated in India in 2006 with a view to creating more wage employment in rural areas thereby ameliorating rural poverty. With the right based framework and demand-driven approach, its initial target has been to guarantee at least 100 days of employment to adults of the rural households every year. But after the completion of more than a decade, the effects and roles of the scheme are found to be manifolds. Particularly, if we consider the impact of women participation under the scheme the results can be witnessed in varied fields. As the scheme has converted some of the unpaid hours of the women into paid hours it has started to change their role in the family. By putting cash in the hands of women MGNREGA has allowed them greater bargaining power in the family thereby diversifying the contributions that women have been making to households. There have been drastic changes in the family consumption pattern as well as family budgeting. While their contribution to the health account has augmented economic security, their role as a financier of the children for their education has led to substantial changes, even impacting the school dropout rate to some extent. All these issues have been taken care of in this chapter based on a micro-level survey done in the district of Nadia, West Bengal.

Chapter 3 - The present study was undertaken to assess age trends in anthropometric measures and nutritional status among adult Mahali females. It was a community-based cross-sectional study, carried out in selected four villages of Bankura district, West Bengal, India. A total of 118 Mahali tribals, aged over 18 years were included in the authors' study. The participants were further classified into three age groups: $\leq 30$ years, 31-49 years, $\geq 50$ years. Anthropometric variables included height, weight, sitting height, knee height, mid-upper arm, medial calf circumferences and body mass index (BMI). In general, an inverse age trend was observed in all these anthropometric variables. This age trend was statistically significant ($p < 0.05$) in case of height, weight, sitting height and medial calf circumference. In nutritional assessment, 75 individuals were found to have chronic energy deficiency (CED). This could have serious health implications.

In: West Bengal
Editor: Rhianu Bowell

ISBN: 978-1-53619-237-7
© 2021 Nova Science Publishers, Inc.

*Chapter 1*

# LIFESTYLE INDUCED ADDICTIVE HABITS: A SOCIO-PHYSIOLOGICAL ISSUE OF KOLKATA, WEST BENGAL

*Gouriprosad Datta[1,\*], PhD, Anurupa Sen[2], PhD, Moumita Das[1], PhD and Subhashree Basu[3], PhD*

[1]Department of Physiology, Rammohan College, Kolkata, West Bengal, India
[2]Department of Physiology, City College, Kolkata, West Bengal, India
[3]Department of Physiology, Tamralipta Mahavidyalaya, Tamluk, Purba Medinipur, West Bengal, India

## ABSTRACT

Globally, industrialization and urbanization are leading to improvement in society's economic condition which is often accompanied by lifestyle changes including physical inactivity, unhealthy diet and harmful use of tobacco and alcohol. These altered lifestyles bring about non-communicable diseases (NCDs) like obesity, hypertension

---

[\*] Corresponding Author's E-mail: dattagp@yahoo.co.in.

(HTN) and diabetes mellitus (DM). The risk factors of the lifestyle induced NCDs are measurable and largely modifiable. So, continuous surveillance on the levels and patterns of risk factors is of fundamental importance to control NCDs.

The study was conducted on 1216 male individuals of different socio-economic status residing at Kolkata, West Bengal, with age ranged 20–60 years. WHO STEP-wise tool was used for face-to-face interviews and a suitably modified WHO-NCD risk factor questionnaire was employed. Personal information regarding physical activity, smoking, smokeless tobacco (SLT) and alcohol consumption along with the personal and family history of HTN and DM were recorded. All the physiological and anthropometric variables were measured using standard procedures. The cutoff values provided by WHO, JNC-VII and ADA were used to classify obesity, HTN and DM, respectively. Different body composition analysis and somatotyping were also done. All statistical computations were performed with SPSS 20.0. For all analyses, $p < 0.05$ were considered as statistically significant.

Smoking, SLT use, alcohol consumption and physical inactivity were observed among 39.1%, 26.7%, 30% and 72.9% people, respectively. Current smokers had increased heart rate (HR), systolic blood pressure (SBP), diastolic blood pressure (DBP) and random blood sugar (RBS) values whereas body mass index (BMI) and waist circumference (WC) decreased with increase in number of cigarettes smoked/day. The increase in drinking quantity significantly increased SBP, DBP, WC and waist-hip ratio (WHR) values. RBS was the highest among light drinkers whereas BMI was the highest among heavy drinkers. Highest DBP and SBP value were observed in 'Alcoholic' and 'Smoker-Alcoholic' group, respectively. 'Smoker-Alcoholic' group had highest mean value of RBS and lowest value was noticed in 'Alcoholic' group. BMI, WC and WHR were also significantly higher in 'Alcoholic' group. All skinfold (SKF) thicknesses, muscle girths, percent body fat (%BF), fat mass (FM), percent muscle mass (%MM), muscle mass (MM), endomorphy and mesomorphy rating decreased with increase in cigarettes smoked/day while ectomorphy rating showed a reverse trend. All the muscle girths, bone widths, skeletal mass (SM), MM, abdominal SKF, FM and lean body mass (LBM) values showed a linear increasing pattern with increase in alcohol consumption whereas subscapular and mid-thigh SKFs showed a decreasing trend. Moreover, all the alcoholics were mesomorphic endomorph. Highest mean values of FM and LBM were found in the 'Alcoholic' group. They also had higher MM, percent skeletal mass (%SM) and SM. Additionally, 'Alcoholics were less ectomorphic, 'Smokers were less mesomorphic and 'Smoker-alcoholics were less endomorphic.

The changed lifestyle demonstrated severe impact on prevalence of NCDs and they also significantly changed the anthropometric and body composition parameters as well as the somatotype ratings. Avoidance to addiction and changes in lifestyle could be an important intervention in preventing/delaying the ongoing upswing in prevalence of NCDs and their associated risk factors.

**Keywords:** addiction, alcohol consumption, lifestyle diseases, non-communicable diseases, smoking, smokeless tobacco, soamtotype

## INTRODUCTION

Lifestyle often describes "The way people live" reflecting a whole range of social values, attitudes, activities and the upcoming stress factors (Thompson et al., 1982). With the advancement in the society, along with scientific and technological progress, there has been a dramatic shift in the way human beings are leading their lives which is sometimes referred as modern way of living (Chakma & Gupta, 2014). "Lifestyle diseases" are associated with the manner a person or group of people lives on a daily basis. In other words, lifestyle diseases characterize those diseases whose occurrences are primarily based on the daily habits of people and are a result of an inappropriate relationship of people with their environment. These diseases are non-communicable and become more widespread as countries grow to be industrialized and people tend to be more mechanized. The onset of these diseases is insidious; they take years to develop and once encountered do not lead themselves easily to cure. These are different from other diseases because they are potentially preventable and can be lowered with changes in diet, lifestyle and environment. In the second half of the 20$^{th}$ century, people's diet changed substantially with the increased consumption of meat, dairy products, vegetable oils, processed food etc. These alterations in food habits along with lifestyle changes such as reduction in physical activities, consumption of alcohol and SLT consumption, increased smoking habit etc. have resulted in high prevalence of NCDs. These diseases include HTN, heart disease, stroke, obesity, DM and, diseases associated with smoking and alcohol abuse such as tobacco induced cancers, chronic bronchitis, emphysema, alcoholic liver disease and premature mortality (Chakma & Gupta, 2014).

Lifestyle related disorders are leading causes of ill-health in developing and developed countries and therefore the above area demands research work to be undertaken. Hiking in economic status and standard of living has also contributed to alterations in lifestyle patterns. The sedentary nature of job compounded with wrong choice of food along with irregular dietary pattern and addictive habits lead to obesity among people of different age groups. The situation is alarming for India and the drastically changing lifestyle pattern of Kolkata, the state capital of West Bengal, also cannot be overlooked in this regard.

Available survey reports made their comments only on socio-economic status (SES), geographical location etc., but only few reports are available regarding the physiological or pathological conditions of the population surveyed at least in urban areas, among the male individuals of Kolkata, in particular. So, the present study comprises not only the changes in cardiovascular and physiological parameters, but also to find out any significant alteration in body fat distribution pattern, changes in body musculature, bone health and somatotype with smoking and alcohol separately, and in combination, as these two have devastating effects on almost every organ system of our body. This is one of the most sensitive areas that should be given focus.

## METHOD

### Selection of Subjects

The survey based cross sectional study was conducted among randomly selected 1500 male individuals of central Kolkata, West Bengal, India. Among them 18.93% (n = 284) people were excluded from the study due to presence of either physical disability or based on medical history such as any major surgery, pacemaker insertion, and cerebral or cardiac stroke and due to missing values of several parameters. Finally, 1216 individuals were included in the study. The study was conducted for a period of 12 months starting from October 2015 to December 2016. The age range of the study population was 20-60 years. Individuals of different designations with various job types were included in this study after obtaining necessary permission from their competent authorities. A self-structured questionnaire was designed for the purpose of data collection which includes all the details about socio-demographic and personal history.

**Study Design**

For the present study, face-to-face interviews using questions based on the WHO STEP-wise tool (WHO, 2013) was used and the WHO-NCD risk factor questionnaire was suitably modified. Information on socio-demographic variables and lifestyle related NCD risk factors (tobacco use, alcohol use and physical activity) as well as information regarding the personal and family history of HTN and DM were also included. For data collection, the subjects were requested to make an appointment, and measurements were made at their respective working place during their free time.

**Ethical Clearance**

This noninvasive study was approved by the "Institutional Ethics Committee for Biomedical Research involving Human Subjects, Rammohan College," constituted in accordance to the guidelines framed by Indian Council of Medical Research. Written consent was obtained from each participant to act as volunteers in the study without any support in terms of cash or kind. The content and purpose of the study, the methods to be followed, the risks, and the potential benefits of the study were clearly explained to the participants. After getting written consent from individuals and permission from their authorities, subjects were requested to make an appointment and measurements were made at their respective working place or home (whichever is nearer) during their free time.

## Evaluation of SES

Depending on the modified "Kuppuswamy's Socioeconomic Status Scale" (Shaikh & Pathak, 2017) the subjects were classified as belonging to upper SES if the total score is 26–29, middle SES (upper middle and lower middle) if the total score is 11–25 and lower SES (upper lower and lower) if the total score is <11.

## Evaluation of Educational Status

Primarily the subjects were classified into 7 (seven) groups according to "Kuppuswamy's Socioeconomic Status Scale" (Shaikh & Pathak, 2017), like illiterate, primary school, middle school, high school, intermediate, graduate or post graduate and profession or honors. For analysis, above mentioned groups were merged into three groups: Lower education (people either illiterate or completed primary school and middle school), Moderate education (completed high school or Intermediate) and Higher education (having graduate or post graduate and profession or honors degree).

## Classification of Smokers

For the present study, smokers were classified as non-smoker (if they have not smoked ever), light smoker (who smoke 1-9 cigarettes or bidis/day), moderate smoker (who smoke 10-19 cigarettes or bidis/day), heavy smoker (who smoke >20 cigarettes or bidis/day) and ex-smoker (if they smoked regularly for >6 months but not smoke anymore for last one year).

## Classification of Alcoholics

Alcoholics were grouped into five categories: non- drinker (subjects who had never drink in their lifetime), light drinker (who drank on a daily basis up to 120 ml/day), moderate drinker (who drink 120-300 ml/day), heavy drinker (who drink more than 300 ml/day) and ex-drinker (who previously consumed alcohol but did not consume any alcohol in the previous one year).

## Classification in Accordance with SLT Consumption

SLT consumption was defined as any form of tobacco consumed orally and not smoked. These included moist oral snuff, chewing tobacco and tobacco used with betel quid, areca nut, pan masala. The population was categorized into: *non-users of SLT and SLT users.*

## Classification According to Family History of DM and HTN

Family history of HTN or DM was assessed by a questionnaire method. People were considered with a positive parental history of DM or HTN if their parents or any one of them (father or mother) had a history of DM or HTN.

## Classification According to Physical Activity

Physical activity was assessed by asking about both work-related and leisure-time physical activities. The participants were categorized into two groups:

    a. People regularly involved in exercise i.e., leisure time physical activity > 30 minutes a day and for at least 3 days in a week.

b. People are not involved in regular physical exercise.

## Determination of Different Physiological Parameters

Resting HR was measured from the radial artery for 1 min with the help of stopwatch (Racer, Coimbatore, Tamil Nadu, India). Blood pressure (BP) was measured with standard mercury sphygmomanometer (Life Line, Kolkata, West Bengal, India) and stethoscope (Duo Sonic, Kolkata, West Bengal, India) after the participants had rested for 5 min (Perloff, 1993). At least two readings at 5-min interval were recorded, and if a high BP (>140/90 mm Hg) was noted, a third reading was taken after 30 min. The lowest of the three readings was taken as blood pressure. A person was considered as suffering from HTN if SBP was 140 mm Hg or above and/or DBP 90 mm Hg or above or is already under treatment for HTN (Sen et al., 2015).

Using the Accu-Check Active glucometer, random blood sugar level was recorded in all subjects. Under all aseptic precautions, blood was collected from the fingertip using sterile disposable lancets. The blood drop was then placed on the yellow window of the Accu-Chek sensor test strip whose electrode was then inserted into the glucometer and the reading obtained. DM was reported if the RBS level was ≥ 200 mg/dL according to the classification provided by American Diabetes Association (ADA) where random means at any time of the day without regard to time since last meal or taking any anti-diabetic drug (ADA. 2016).

## Determination of Different Anthropometric Parameters

Body height and body weight were measured to the nearest 0.1 cm and 0.1 kg by an anthropometric rod and portable weighing machine (Advanced Technocracy, Ambala City, Haryana, India), respectively, with the subjects standing barefoot and in light clothing. The BMI was calculated as weight (kg) BMI >23.0 and >25.0 kg/m$^2$ was taken as cut off value for overweight and obesity, respectively (WHO, 2000). The WC was measured at the midpoint between the inferior border of the subcostal margin and iliac crest in the midaxillary line after normal expiration in standing posture; the hip circumference (HC) was measured at the widest part of the hip across both greater trochanters, from which the WHR was calculated. Truncal obesity was diagnosed when WHR was >0.90 and abdominal obesity, when WC was >90 cm in men (WHO, 2000). Another obesity parameter, waist-to-height ratio (WHtR) was calculated by WC (cm)/ height (cm). Individuals having value of WHtR ≥ 0.50 was considered as obese (Ashwell & Gibson, 2016).

## Determination of Body Density (BD) and %BF Using SKF Thickness

Several SKF thicknesses (Biceps, Triceps, Subscapular, Suprailiac, Abdominal, Mid-thigh and Mid-calf SKF) were measured by using Harpenden skinfold caliper following standard procedure. BD was estimated from Biceps, Triceps, Subscapular and Suprailiac SKFs using the Durnin and Womersley equation (Durnin & Womersley, 1974) which was validated in Asian Indians (Kuriyan et al., 1998) and from BD, %BF was computed in accordance to Siri's equation (Siri, 1956). FM and LBM were also calculated.

The following equations were used for the present study:

For men, BD = $1.1715 - 0.0779 \times \log_{10}$ (Biceps + Triceps + Subscapular + Suprailiac)
%BF = $(4.95/BD - 4.5) \times 100$
FM (kg) = $(\%BF/100) \times$ Weight (kg)
LBM (kg) = Weight (kg) − FM (kg)

## Determination of MM and %MM

Forearm, Upper arm, Thigh and Calf girths were measured by a non-stretching measuring tape following standard procedure The MM and regional muscularity of the subjects were estimated using the formula proposed by Martin et al., (1990). %MM was calculated from the obtained value of MM. The equation is as follows:

MM (kg) = (ht × (0.0553CTG$^2$ + 0.0987FG$^2$ + 0.0331CCG$^2$) – 2445) × 0.001

where: ht is stature in cm,
CTG is corrected thigh girth = thigh girth – π (front thigh SKF/10),
FG is maximum forearm girth,
CCG is corrected calf girth = calf girth – π (medial calf SKF/10)
%MM = (MM kg /body mass) × 100

## Determination of SM and %SM

Following standard procedure different bone diameters (Wrist, Humerus, Femur and Ankle) were measured using sliding caliper. SM was then calculated by Drinkwater et al., (1986) equation. After calculating the SM, %SM was also computed. The equation is as follows:

SM (kg) = ((humerus + wrist + femur + ankle)/4)$^2$ × height × 0.92 × 0.001
%SM = (SM / body mass) × 100

## Determination of Anthropometric Somatotype

By using Heath Carter Somatotypes method (Carter & Heath, 1990), ten anthropometric measurements were taken which were as follows: i) Standing height, ii) Body weight, iii) Biepicondylar humerus diameter, iv)

Biepicondylar femur diameter, v) Biceps muscle girth, vi) Calf muscle girth, vii) Triceps SKF, viii) Subscapular SKF, ix) Supraspinale SKF and x) Medial calf SKF. Each indicator was measured twice and the average was taken. All three components of somatotypes were calculated with the following formulae:

*Endomorphy* = - 0.7182 + 0.1451 (X) - 0.00068 ($X^2$) + 0.0000014 ($X^3$)

where X = (sum of triceps, subscapular and supraspinale SKFs) multiplied by (170.18/height in cm).

*Mesomorphy* = 0.858 x humerus breadth + 0.601 x femur breadth + 0.188 x corrected arm girth + 0.161 x corrected calf girth − height 0.131 + 4.5.

*Ectomorphy* =Three different equations are used to calculate ectomorphy according to the height-weight Ratio (HWR):

If HWR is greater than or equal to 40.75 then Ectomorphy = 0.732 HWR - 28.58

If HWR is less than 40.75 but greater than 38.25 then Ectomorphy = 0.463 HWR - 17.63

If HWR is equal to or less than 38.25 then Ectomorphy = 0.1

## Somatotype Categories

The different categories of somatotype proposed by Heath-Carter (Carter & Heath, 1990) were simplified into three larger categories:

*Endomorph*: Endomorphy is dominant; mesomorphy and ectomorphy is more than one-half unit lower.

*Mesomorph*: Mesomorphy is dominant; endomorphy and ectomorphy are more than one-half unit lower.

*Ectomorph*: Ectomorphy is dominant; endomorphy and mesomorphy are more than one-half units lower.

## Statistical Analysis

Data was entered using Microsoft excel and analyzed using Statistical Package for Social Sciences software (SPSS, version 20.0). The mean and its corresponding standard error (SE) of mean were computed for continuous variables and frequencies and percentages for categorical variables. Chi square test was used to test the association between categorical variables and independent sample t-test was used to compare means of continuous variables. For all analyses, $p < 0.05$ was considered statistically significant.

## RESULTS

### Socio-Demographic and Lifestyle Characteristic of the Population

A total of 1216 healthy male individuals of Kolkata were studied in this survey based cross-sectional study. The age range of the study population is 20-60 years, having a mean age of 42.56 years. The socio-demographic and lifestyle related information of the study population were described elsewhere (Sen et al., 2016).

### Effect of Different Addictive Habits

*Comparison of physiological and anthropometric parameters, prevalence of NCD risk factors and NCDs among different smoking categories:*

Table 1 shows the comparison of physiological and anthropometric variables among the different smoking categories. It was noticed that ex-smokers were aged and weighed more than non-smokers and current smokers.

**Table 1. Comparison of physiological and anthropometric parameters among different smoking categories**

| Variable | Smoking habit | | | | |
|---|---|---|---|---|---|
| | Non-smoker (n = 634) | Light smoker (n = 233) | Moderate smoker (n = 126) | Heavy smoker (n = 116) | Ex-smoker (n = 107) |
| Age (years)* | 42.24 ± 0.423 | 41.81 ± 0.720 | 42.99 ± 0.930 | 41.99 ± 0.984 | 46.23 ± 1.029 |
| Height (cm) | 168.31 ± 0.289 | 168.31 ± 0.449 | 169.53 ± 0.631 | 167.77 ± 0.662 | 169.05 ± 0.681 |
| Weight (kg) | 66.82 ± 0.437 | 66.44 ± 0.729 | 66.56 ± 1.01 | 64.54 ± 1.03 | 67.36 ± 1.02 |
| HR (beats/min) | 76.70 ± 0.315 | 76.78 ± 0.584 | 77.16 ± 0.763 | 76.45 ± 0.789 | 77.31 ± 0.783 |
| SBP (mm Hg) | 128.44 ± 0.549 | 126.88 ± 0.959 | 127.79 ± 1.42 | 130.0 ± 1.38 | 127.74 ± 1.20 |
| DBP (mm Hg) | 80.92 ± 0.288 | 80.45 ± 0.507 | 80.37 ± 0.776 | 80.72 ± 0.859 | 80.30 ± 0.714 |
| RBS (mg/dL) | 131.80 ± 2.092 | 134.63 ± 3.61 | 135.06 ± 5.04 | 133.43 ± 4.58 | 141.68 ± 7.08 |
| BMI (kg/m$^2$) | 23.52 ± 0.127 | 23.41 ± 0.225 | 23.09 ± 0.299 | 22.89 ± 0.317 | 23.49 ± 0.276 |
| WC (cm) | 90.03 ± 0.391 | 89.61 ± 0.691 | 89.51 ± 0.951 | 88.25 ± 1.06 | 91.54 ± 0.911 |
| WHR | 0.98 ± 0.002 | 0.97 ± 0.004 | 0.98 ± 0.006 | 0.97 ± 0.007 | 0.99 ± 0.005 |
| WHtR | 0.53 ± 0.002 | 0.53 ± 0.004 | 0.53 ± 0.005 | 0.53 ± 0.006 | 0.54 ± 0.005 |

Data were represented as Mean ± SE. * denotes statistical significance.

Among the current smokers, heavy smokers have less weight. HR, SBP and DBP values did not show any significant variation among the different categories. Increased HR was observed among moderate smokers and ex-smokers. Heavy smokers had the highest SBP and DBP values and these values decreased for the ex-smokers. Current smokers had increased RBS values when compared with non-smokers, whereas ex-smokers had the highest mean values of RBS. BMI and WC values showed the same trend where non-smokers and ex-smokers had higher values in comparison to current smokers. BMI and WC values were decreased with an increase in the number of cigarettes/bidis smoked per day and the decrease was highest among heavy smokers. WHR and WHtR values remained almost the same among all the categories but for both the variables ex-smokers had the highest means.

The prevalence of different NCD risk factors among the smoking categories was presented in Figure 1. It was revealed that SLT consumption was significantly higher among ex-smokers and non-smokers whereas current smokers had lower addiction for SLT. People, smoked greater number of cigarettes/bidis per day, were less physically active and it was also observed that highest percentage of heavy smokers were physically inactive. Non-smokers and ex-smokers belong to almost the same activity level. The positive family history of HTN and DM were mostly prevalent among moderate and light smokers, respectively. Alcohol consumption (light, moderate and heavy drinking) was found to be significantly higher among the current smokers in comparison to ex-smokers and non-smokers whereas ex-smokers were mostly ex-drinkers.

From Figure 2, it can be seen that the prevalence of overweight was highest among heavy smokers in comparison to non-smokers and ex-smokers. The prevalence of all the obesity parameters was higher among non-smokers and ex-smokers whereas the increase in smoking cigarettes/bidis per day decreased the prevalence of obesity. When compared with other categories, HTN was observed to be higher among heavy smokers and ex-smokers whereas moderate and ex-smokers had a higher prevalence of DM.

*Lifestyle Induced Addictive Habits* 15

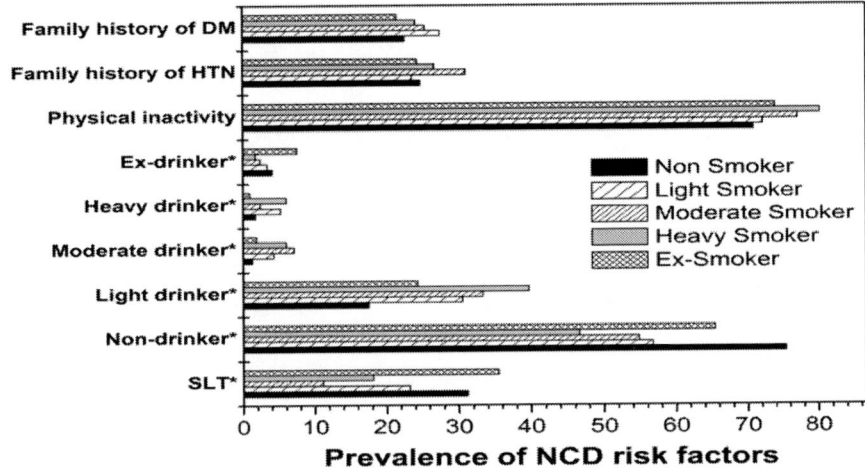

Figure 1. Prevalence of NCD risk factors among different smoking categories.
NCD: Non-communicable diseases; SLT: Smokeless tobacco; HTN: Hypertension;
DM: Diabetes Mellitus. (* denotes statistical significance).

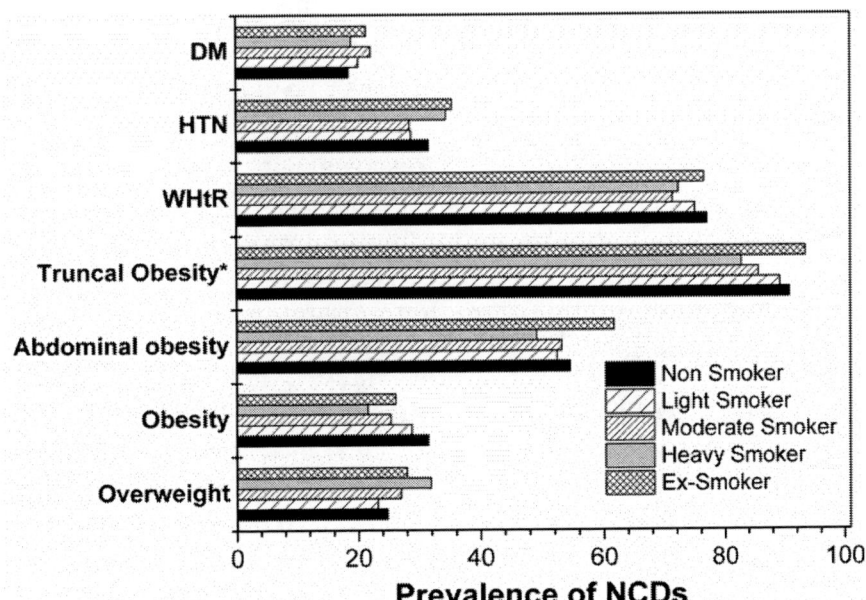

Figure 2. Prevalence of NCDs among different smoking categories.
NCD: Non-communicable diseases; HTN: Hypertension; DM: Diabetes Mellitus.
(* denotes statistical significance).

*Comparison of physiological and anthropometric parameters, prevalence of NCD risk factors and NCDs among different alcoholic categories:*

Table 2 shows that the increase in drinking quantity significantly increases height, weight, SBP, DBP, WC and WHR having the highest mean value among heavy drinkers followed by moderate and light drinkers. These values were quite low in the case of non-drinkers. It was seen that moderate drinkers were aged more. RBS' values were found to be highest among light drinkers. The BMI value was highest among heavy drinkers, whereas WHtR values remained the same for all the categories. The mean values decreased among ex-drinkers, which indicated that quitting drinking habits improved the physiological and anthropometric mean values.

The majority of the ex-smokers were SLT consumers and this addiction was also higher among current drinkers (Figure 3). The sedentary lifestyle was mostly prevalent among heavy drinkers whereas the physical inactivity level was nearly the same among other categories. The family history of HTN and DM was also prevalent among heavy drinkers and moderate drinkers, respectively. In the present investigation, it was observed that ex-alcoholics were ex-smokers. It was also noted that addiction towards smoking increases with an increase in drinking quantity.

Figure 4 shows the prevalence of different NCDs among the alcoholic categories. Prevalence of overweight was the highest among the ex-drinkers in comparison to others. Heavy drinkers were mostly obese. Abdominal obesity increases with increase in drinking quantity being highest among heavy drinkers whereas truncal obesity was mostly prevalent among moderate drinkers. A similar increasing pattern was also observed for WHtR where obesity was mostly prevalent among heavy drinkers. Among the current drinkers, HTN and DM were prevalent among heavy drinkers and light drinkers, respectively.

## Table 2. Comparison of physiologic and anthropometric parameters among different alcoholic categories

| Variable | Alcohol consumption | | | | |
|---|---|---|---|---|---|
| | Non-drinker (n = 803) | Light drinker (n = 296) | Moderate drinker (n = 36) | Heavy drinker (n = 34) | Ex-drinker (n = 47) |
| Age (years) | 42.67 ± 0.39 | 41.86 ± 0.611 | 44.14 ± 1.35 | 43.68 ± 0.958 | 43.11 ± 1.63 |
| Height (cm)* | 168.04 ± 0.256 | 168.78 ± 0.389 | 171.93 ± 1.07 | 171.52 ± 1.13 | 168.57 ± 1.14 |
| Weight (kg)* | 65.87 ± 0.384 | 67.60 ± 0.646 | 68.94 ± 1.98 | 71.45 ± 1.98 | 66.30 ± 1.58 |
| HR (beats/min)* | 76.58 ± 0.299 | 76.66 ± 0.445 | 81.0 ± 1.68 | 79.53 ± 1.07 | 76.09 ± 1.01 |
| SBP (mm Hg)* | 126.81 ± 0.467 | 128.56 ± 0.822 | 138.56 ± 3.23 | 141.06 ± 3.26 | 131.53 ± 2.04 |
| DBP (mm Hg)* | 79.98 ± 0.27 | 81.58 ± 0.391 | 82.89 ± 1.67 | 86.59 ± 1.31 | 81.49 ± 1.45 |
| RBS (mg/dL) | 133.49 ± 1.99 | 137.86 ± 3.34 | 122.39 ± 5.31 | 135.65 ± 6.32 | 118.55 ± 6.68 |
| BMI kg/m$^2$) | 23.27 ± 0.114 | 23.69 ± 0.195 | 23.29 ± 0.598 | 24.23 ± 0.573 | 23.22 ± 0.423 |
| WC (cm)* | 89.17 ± 0.352 | 90.96 ± 0.607 | 92.10 ± 1.57 | 93.35 ± 1.83 | 90.52 ± 1.68 |
| WHR* | 0.97 ± 0.002 | 0.98 ± 0.004 | 0.99 ± 0.008 | 0.99 ± 0.01 | 0.98 ± 0.01 |
| WHtR | 0.53 ± 0.002 | 0.54 ± 0.003 | 0.54 ± 0.009 | 0.54 ± 0.009 | 0.54 ± 0.009 |

Data were represented as Mean ± SE. * denotes statistical significance.

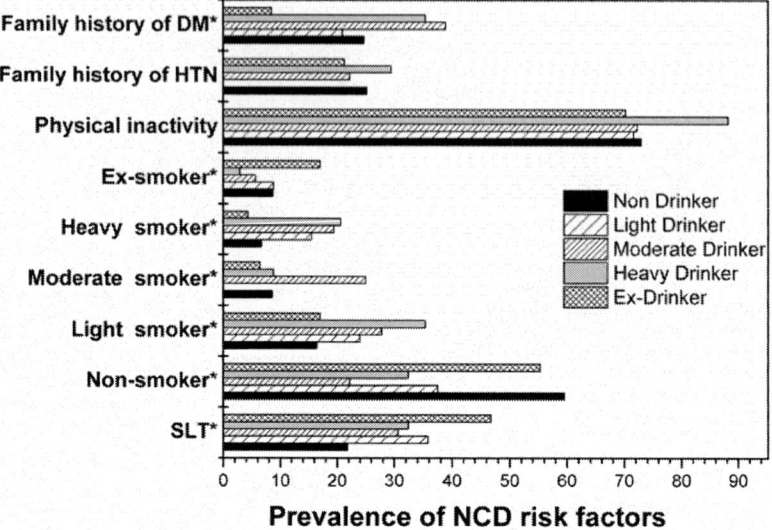

Figure 3. Prevalence of NCD risk factors among different alcoholic categories.
NCD: Non-communicable diseases; SLT: Smokeless tobacco; HTN: Hypertension;
DM: Diabetes Mellitus. (* denotes statistical significance).

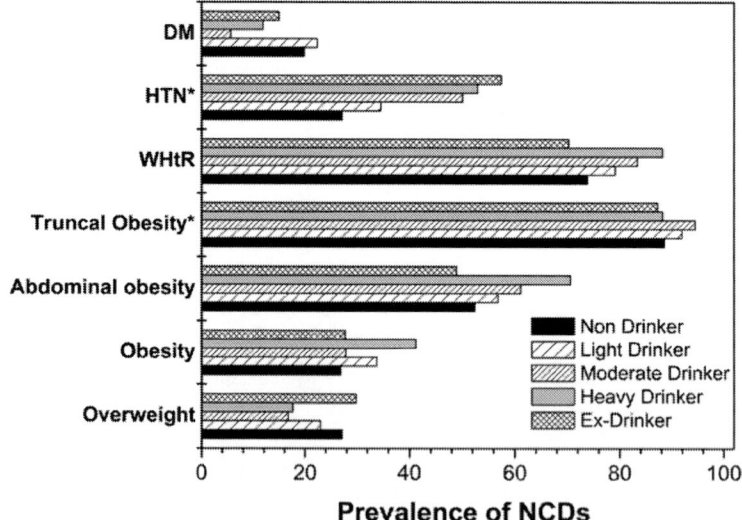

Figure 4. Prevalence of NCDs among different alcoholic categories.
NCD: Non-communicable diseases; HTN: Hypertension; DM: Diabetes Mellitus.
(* denotes statistical significance).

*Comparative analysis of physiological and anthropometric parameters, NCD risk factors and prevalence of NCDs among different addictive groups:*

In the previous segments, we distinguished the individual effect of smoking and alcohol consumption on different physiological, anthropometric parameters as well as prevalence of NCD risk factors and NCDs. Now to find out the effect of smoking and drinking only as well as their combination, the whole study population was further divided into four major groups:

- Nonsmoker–Nonalcoholic (NS–NA): people in this group were not addicted to either smoking or alcohol.
- Only smoker (S): people were addicted only to smoking tobacco but not to alcohol.
- Only alcoholic (A): people were addicted only to alcohol but not to tobacco.
- Smoker–Alcoholic (S–A): people were addicted to both tobacco smoking and alcohol.

Among the study people, 48.8% were not addicted to cigarette or alcohol, 21.4% were only addicted to cigarette/bidi, 12.2% consume alcohol and another 17.6% were addicted to both smoking and alcohol.

Significant alterations were noted in all the physiological and anthropometric parameters (Table 3), except HR, RBS, BMI and WHtR, when compared among different addictive habit groups by ANOVA. It was observed that 'A' group had highest mean value of height while 'NS–NA' group had lowest. 'A' group also gained maximum weight and the 'S' group significantly lose their weight. Lowest value of HR was observed in 'NS–NA' group and highest in 'A' group, but this difference remained statistically non–significant. Similar result persists for DBP where highest DBP value was noticed in 'A' group.

## Table 3. Comparative analysis of different Physiological and Anthropometric parameters, Prevalence of NCD risk factors and NCDs among different addictive groups

| Variables | Addictive Habits | | | |
|---|---|---|---|---|
| | NS-NA (n = 594) | S (n = 260) | A (n = 148) | S-A (n = 214) |
| Height (cm)* | 167.98 ± 0.302 | 168.17 ± 0.438 | 169.52 ± 0.560 | 169.35 ± 0.459 |
| Weight (kg)* | 66.06 ± 0.425 | 65.58± 0.743 | 68.43 ± 0.998 | 67.80 ± 0.734 |
| HR (beats/min) | 76.48 ± 0.336 | 76.69 ± 0.545 | 77.49 ± 0.603 | 77.31 ± 0.570 |
| SBP (mm Hg)* | 127.47± 0.551 | 126.15 ± 0.804 | 130.41 ± 1.126 | 130.98 ± 1.178 |
| DBP (mm Hg)* | 80.11 ± 0.308 | 80.08 ± 0.527 | 82.16 ± 0.498 | 82.09 ± 0.549 |
| RBS (mg/dL) | 132.64 ± 2.190 | 133.98 ± 3.838 | 130.28 ± 3.783 | 138.70 ± 3.972 |
| WC (cm)* | 89.43 ± 0.385 | 88.85 ± 0.714 | 91.92 ± 0.909 | 90.85 ± 0.681 |
| WHR* | 0.97 ± 0.002 | 0.97 ± 0.004 | 0.99 ± 0.005 | 0.98 ± 0.004 |
| BMI (kg/m2) | 23.35 ± 0.121 | 23.14 ± 0.230 | 23.72 ± 0.277 | 23.63 ± 0.233 |
| WHtR | 0.53 ± 0.002 | 0.53 ± 0.004 | 0.54 ± 0.005 | 0.54 ± 0.004 |
| Physical inactivity | 71.04 (422) | 76.92 (200) | 68.92 (102) | 75.7 (162) |
| Smokeless tobacco consumption* | 24.41 (145) | 20 (52) | 39.19 (58) | 32.71 (70) |
| Overweight* | 27.27 (162) | 26.92 (70) | 17.57 (26) | 25.23 (54) |
| Obesity* | 28.28 (168) | 24.62 (64) | 37.84 (56) | 29.91 (64) |
| Abdominal obesity | 52.53 (312) | 51.54 (134) | 62.16 (92) | 56.07 (120) |
| Truncal obesity | 89.56 (532) | 86.15 (224) | 93.24 (138) | 90.65 (194) |
| Waist to Height Ratio* | 75.08 (446) | 70.78 (184) | 81.08 (120) | 79.44 (170) |
| Hypertension* | 29.63 (176) | 26.92 (70) | 40.54 (60) | 35.51 (76) |
| Diabetes Mellitus | 20.88 (124) | 17.69 (46) | 14.86 (22) | 21.5 (46) |

Data were represented as Mean ± SE and n (%). * denotes statistical significance.

Significantly lower DBP value was observed in 'S' group when compared with 'A' group (Table 3). 'A' significantly increased SBP value in 'S–A' group compared to 'S' group and 'NS–NA' group was also noted. Moreover, for both SBP and DBP values, 'NS–NA' and 'S' groups had lower mean values and 'S–A' and 'A' groups had higher mean values. These results indicate that alcohol itself can increase blood pressure in people who are addicted to only alcohol and both-smoking and alcohol. 'S–A' group had highest mean value of RBS and lowest value was noticed in 'A' group which suggest that, alcohol exert some protective action in alcoholics. Abdominal obesity was significantly higher in 'A' group compared to 'NS–NA' and 'S' groups. When compared among the groups, 'S' group had the lowest value of WC. Similar pattern was also noted in WHR where the 'A' group had significantly increased mean value in comparison to 'NS–NA' and 'S' groups. 'S' group had lowest 'BMI' value while highest value was found in 'A' group. Again, 'S–A' group had BMI value lower than 'A' group but greater than 'S' group whereas 'NS–NA' group had higher value than 'S' group. WHtR value in 'A' and 'S–A' groups were same and a similar result was obtained showing equal WHtR value in 'S' and 'NS–NA' groups.

As observed from Table 3, highest prevalence of physical inactivity persists among the smokers, followed by 'S–A' group, 'NS–NA' and 'A' group. 39.19%, 32.71%, 24.41% and 20% people of the 'A,' 'S–A,' 'NS–NA' and 'S' group were addicted to SLT, respectively. It was interesting to observe that prevalence of overall body adiposity, abdominal obesity, truncal obesity and WHtR were higher among the people of 'A' group, followed by 'S–A,' 'NS–NA' group and the lowest prevalence was observed among the 'S' group. A similar trend was also observed for the prevalence of HTN. DM was prevalent among 21.5% of 'A' group, followed by 20.88% in 'NS–NA' group, 17.69% in 'S' group and 14.86 % in 'S–A' group.

Effect of different addictive habits on body composition and somatotype components:

*Comparison of body composition and somatotype components among different smoking categories:*

Table 4 shows the differences in body composition and somatotype components among different smoking categories. In comparison to non-smokers, thickness of all the SKFs, %BF and FM decreased in a liner fashion with increase in number of cigarettes smoked per day, whereas smoking cessation increased all the SKF values, %BF and FM. Similar linear decreasing trend was also observed for all muscle girths, %MM and MM among the smokers. On the other hand, quitting smoking improved muscle girth and MM. In comparison to non-smokers, wrist and humerus bone widths slightly increased among light and moderate smokers, but showed reduction in heavy smokers. Femur width showed a decreasing pattern with increase in smoking habit. In case of ankle width, light and heavy smokers had lower values than non-smokers, whereas moderate smokers had a greater width. %SM increased with increase in number of cigarettes. SM also increased among light and moderate smokers but decreased among heavy smokers. When compared with non-smokers, endomorphy and mesomorphy ratings showed a linear decreasing trend with increasing smoking pattern whereas ectomorphy rating showed a reverse trend. Ex-smokers had more or less similar ratings to non-smokers.

*Comparison of body composition and somatotype components among different alcoholic categories:*

Comparison of various body composition and somatotype components among different alcohol consumption categories were represented in Table 5. Compared to non-alcoholics, biceps, triceps, suprailiac SKFs and %BF increased among light and heavy drinkers but lowered among moderate drinkers. Subscapular and mid-thigh SKFs decreased with an increase in drinking frequency. Abdominal SKF, FM and LBM values showed a linear increasing pattern with an increase in drinking alcohol. Except thigh girth and %MM, current alcoholics also had higher mean values of all the muscle girths and MM. Similar to muscle girths, bone widths and SM also increased with increase in alcohol consumption. All the alcoholics showed mesomorphic endomorph somatotypes. Compared to non-drinkers, endomorphy ratings decreased among current drinkers. Mesomorphy ratings increased among light drinkers whereas moderate and heavy drinkers had lower values. Ectomorphy rating decreased among light and heavy drinkers, whereas moderate drinkers were more ectomorphic.

**Table 4. Comparison of body composition and somatotype components among different smoking categories**

| Variables | Smoking habit | | | | |
|---|---|---|---|---|---|
| | Non-smoker (n = 634) | Light smoker (n = 233) | Moderate smoker (n = 126) | Heavy smoker (n = 116) | Ex-smoker (n = 107) |
| **SKF Thickness** | | | | | |
| Biceps * (mm) | 6.80 ± 0.11 | 6.49 ± 0.19 | 6.39 ± 0.23 | 6.06 ± 0.28 | 7.10 ± 0.26 |
| Triceps (mm) | 10.11 ± 0.15 | 9.88 ± 0.23 | 9.58 ± 0.32 | 9.45 ± 0.36 | 10.03 ± 0.34 |
| Subscapular (mm) | 21.41 ± 0.32 | 20.86 ± 0.53 | 20.68 ± 0.69 | 20.43 ± 0.84 | 21.59 ± 0.71 |
| Suprailiac (mm) | 21.24 ± 0.34 | 20.51 ± 0.62 | 20.36 ± 0.78 | 18.80 ± 0.87 | 20.9 ± 0.80 |
| Abdomen (mm) | 33.64 ± 0.43 | 32.98 ± 0.76 | 32.76 ± 1.02 | 31.14 ± 1.17 | 34.61 ± 0.99 |
| Mid-thigh * (mm) | 14.89 ± 0.19 | 14.20 ± 0.33 | 14.7 ± 0.41 | 13.18 ± 0.44 | 14.03 ± 0.40 |
| Mid-calf (mm) | 10.70 ± 0.15 | 10.23 ± 0.26 | 10.63 ± 0.33 | 9.76 ± 0.34 | 10.17 ± 0.29 |
| %BF* | 28.05 ± 0.24 | 27.43 ± 0.42 | 27.17 ± 0.56 | 26.27 ± 0.68 | 28.24 ± 0.54 |
| Fat-mass(kg) | 19.24 ± 0.25 | 18.77 ± 0.45 | 18.61 ± 0.59 | 17.59 ± 0.67 | 19.43 ± 0.59 |
| LBM (kg) | 47.59 ± 0.22 | 47.67 ± 0.36 | 47.95 ± 0.54 | 46.95 ± 0.49 | 47.93 ± 0.54 |
| **Muscle girth** | | | | | |
| Forearm (cm) | 25.89 ± 0.08 | 25.85 ± 0.12 | 25.66 ± 0.27 | 25.61 ± 0.18 | 25.95 ± 0.17 |
| Upperarm (cm) | 27.62 ± 0.11 | 27.42 ± 0.18 | 27.18 ± 0.25 | 27.15 ± 0.27 | 27.52 ± 0.23 |
| Thigh* (cm) | 50.19 ± 0.21 | 49.39 ± 0.38 | 49.51 ± 0.5 | 48.51 ± 0.55 | 50.41 ± 0.43 |
| Calf (cm) | 35.14 ± 0.18 | 34.88 ± 0.21 | 34.86 ± 0.36 | 34.38 ± 0.31 | 34.97 ± 0.32 |
| %MM | 25.46 ± 0.18 | 24.94 ± 0.31 | 25.11 ± 0.4 | 24.77 ± 0.37 | 26.04 ± 0.31 |
| MM (kg) | 17.17 ± 0.17 | 16.69 ± 0.29 | 16.81 ± 0.41 | 16.16 ± 0.41 | 17.57 ± 0.34 |
| **Bone width** | | | | | |
| Wrist* (cm) | 5.22 ± 0.01 | 5.24 ± 0.02 | 5.25 ± 0.03 | 5.22 ± 0.03 | 5.33 ± 0.03 |
| Humerous (cm) | 6.45 ± 0.02 | 6.47 ± 0.03 | 6.47 ± 0.04 | 6.42 ± 0.04 | 6.52 ± 0.04 |

## Table 4. (Continued)

| Variable | Smoking habit | | | | |
|---|---|---|---|---|---|
| | Non-smoker (n = 634) | Light smoker (n = 233) | Moderate smoker (n = 126) | Heavy smoker (n = 116) | Ex-smoker (n = 107) |
| Femur (cm) | 9.29 ± 0.03 | 9.28 ± 0.04 | 9.27 ± 0.06 | 9.20 ± 0.06 | 9.44 ± 0.06 |
| Ankle (cm) | 6.80 ± 0.02 | 6.77 ± 0.02 | 6.82 ± 0.05 | 6.74 ± 0.04 | 6.83 ± 0.05 |
| % SM | 11.36 ± 0.06 | 11.46 ± 0.10 | 11.54 ± 0.15 | 11.62 ± 0.16 | 11.59 ± 0.13 |
| SM (kg) | 7.49 ± 0.04 | 7.50 ± 0.06 | 7.60 ± 0.11 | 7.37 ± 0.09 | 7.73 ± 0.10 |
| Somatotype components | | | | | |
| Endomorphy | 5.10 ± 0.06 | 4.95 ± 0.11 | 4.86 ± 0.14 | 4.69 ± 0.17 | 5.10 ± 0.14 |
| Mesomorphy | 4.03 ± 0.05 | 4.01 ± 0.08 | 3.79 ± 0.12 | 3.86 ± 0.13 | 4.07 ± 0.11 |
| Ectomorphy | 2.04 ± 0.05 | 2.11 ± 0.09 | 2.29 ± 0.12 | 2.30 ± 0.15 | 2.04 ± 0.11 |

Data were represented as Mean ± SE. * denotes statistical significance.

**Table 5. Comparison of body composition and somatotype components among different alcohol consumption categories**

| Variable | Alcohol consumption | | | | |
|---|---|---|---|---|---|
| | Non-drinker (n = 803) | Light drinker (n = 296) | Moderate drinker (n = 36) | Heavy drinker (n = 34) | Ex-drinker (n = 47) |
| **SKF Thickness** | | | | | |
| Biceps (mm) | 6.71 ± 0.09 | 6.54 ± 0.17 | 6.48 ± 0.46 | 7.18 ± 0.53 | 6.09 ± 0.36 |
| Triceps (mm) | 9.98 ± 0.13 | 9.83 ± 0.22 | 9.64 ± 0.68 | 10.19 ± 0.8 | 10.0 ± 0.45 |
| Subscapular (mm) | 21.21 ± 0.28 | 20.76 ± 0.47 | 20.62 ± 1.57 | 20.45 ± 1.56 | 21.84 ± 0.96 |
| Suprailiac (mm) | 20.91 ± 0.31 | 20.49 ± 0.52 | 20.11 ± 1.68 | 20.55 ± 1.53 | 20.14 ± 1.09 |
| Abdomen (mm) | 32.96 ± 0.36 | 33.67 ± 0.67 | 34.54 ± 1.9 | 35.09 ± 2.07 | 33.71 ± 1.67 |
| Mid-thigh (mm) | 14.66 ± 0.16 | 14.23 ± 0.29 | 13.99 ± 1.0 | 13.97 ± 0.75 | 14.25 ± 0.56 |
| Mid-calf (mm) | 10.56 ± 0.12 | 10.40 ± 0.25 | 10.62 ± 0.95 | 9.98 ± 0.48 | 9.41 ± 0.45 |
| %BF | 27.83 ± 0.22 | 27.41 ± 0.37 | 26.94 ± 1.18 | 27.23 ± 1.34 | 28.0 ± 0.70 |
| Fat-mass (kg) | 18.33 ± 0.22 | 19.04 ± 0.38 | 19.29 ± 1.33 | 20.16 ± 1.33 | 19.02 ± 0.85 |
| LBM* (kg) | 47.03 ± 0.19 | 48.56 ± 0.26 | 49.65 ± 0.78 | 51.28 ± 0.91 | 47.28 ± 0.81 |
| **Muscle Girth** | | | | | |
| Forearm (cm) | 25.81 ± 0.07 | 25.87 ± 0.17 | 25.98 ± 0.33 | 25.90 ± 0.38 | 25.94 ± 0.26 |
| Upper arm (cm) | 27.38 ± 0.09 | 27.63 ± 0.15 | 28.03 ± 0.52 | 27.82 ± 0.57 | 27.62 ± 0.4 |
| Thigh (cm) | 49.93 ± 0.19 | 49.84 ± 0.33 | 48.60 ± 0.38 | 49.73 ± 0.51 | 49.06 ± 0.82 |
| Calf (cm) | 34.93 ± 0.15 | 35.03 ± 0.18 | 35.05 ± 0.6 | 35.09 ± 0.42 | 35.16 ± 0.6 |
| %MM* | 25.62 ± 0.15 | 25.11 ± 0.25 | 23.68 ± 0.78 | 24.18 ± 0.88 | 24.76 ± 0.82 |
| MM (kg) | 16.96 ± 0.15 | 17.09 ± 0.26 | 16.54 ± 0.81 | 17.46 ± 0.86 | 16.49 ± 0.69 |

## Table 5. (Continued)

| Variables | Alcohol consumption | | | | |
|---|---|---|---|---|---|
| | Non-drinker (n = 803) | Light drinker (n = 296) | Moderate drinker (n = 36) | Heavy drinker (n = 34) | Ex-drinker (n = 47) |
| Bone width | | | | | |
| Wrist* (cm) | 5.22 ± 0.01 | 5.27 ± 0.02 | 5.34 ± 0.05 | 5.32 ± 0.05 | 5.19 ± 0.04 |
| Humerous* (cm) | 6.43 ± 0.02 | 6.51 ± 0.02 | 6.59 ± 0.08 | 6.58 ± 0.08 | 6.47 ± 0.06 |
| Femur *(cm) | 9.27 ± 0.02 | 9.30 ± 0.04 | 9.46 ± 0.11 | 9.56 ± 0.08 | 9.39 ± 0.1 |
| Ankle* (cm) | 6.77 ± 0.02 | 6.80 ± 0.02 | 7.0 ± 0.08 | 6.88 ± 0.08 | 6.91 ± 0.1 |
| % SM | 11.45 ± 0.06 | 11.36 ± 0.09 | 11.75 ± 0.26 | 11.34 ± 0.31 | 11.61 ± 0.18 |
| SM* (kg) | 7.45 ± 0.04 | 7.58 ± 0.06 | 7.98 ± 0.16 | 7.96 ± 0.17 | 7.63 ± 0.17 |
| Somatotype components | | | | | |
| Endomorphy | 5.04 ± 0.05 | 4.93 ± 0.09 | 4.83 ± 0.31 | 4.92 ± 0.32 | 5.07 ± 0.19 |
| Mesomorphy | 3.96 ± 0.04 | 4.05 ± 0.07 | 3.88 ± 0.26 | 3.95 ± 0.19 | 4.13 ± 0.17 |
| Ectomorphy | 2.13 ± 0.05 | 2.02 ± 0.07 | 2.38 ± 0.24 | 1.94 ± 0.22 | 2.13 ± 0.17 |

Data were represented as Mean ± SE. * denotes statistical significance.

**Table 6. Comparison of body composition and somatotype components among Nonsmoker-Nonalcoholic, Only Smoker, Only Alcoholic and Smoker-Alcoholic**

| Variables | Addictive Habits | | | |
|---|---|---|---|---|
| | Non-smoker Non-alcoholic (n = 594) | Smoker (n = 260) | Alcoholic (n = 148) | Smoker –Alcoholic (n = 214) |
| **SKF thickness** | | | | |
| Biceps (mm) | 6.75 ± 0.11 | 6.60 ± 0.18 | 6.94 ± 0.24 | 6.25 ± 0.19 |
| Triceps (mm) | 10.03 ± 0.14 | 9.96 ± 0.22 | 10.0 ± 0.30 | 9.63 ± 0.27 |
| Subscapular (mm) | 21.44 ± 0.31 | 20.90 ± 0.53 | 20.24 ± 0.66 | 20.91 ± 0.58 |
| Suprailiac (mm) | 21.01 ± 0.33 | 20.64 ± 0.59 | 20.89 ± 0.74 | 20.03 ± 0.62 |
| Abdomen (mm) | 33.18 ± 0.43 | 32.75 ± 0.74 | 33.90 ± 0.94 | 33.72 ± 0.81 |
| Mid-thigh (mm) | 14.74 ± 0.18 | 14.51 ± 0.3 | 14.32 ± 0.41 | 13.93 ± 0.35 |
| Mid-calf (mm) | 10.58 ± 0.14 | 10.39 ± 0.22 | 10.44 ± 0.29 | 10.22 ± 0.33 |
| %BF | 28.04 ± 0.246 | 27.48 ± 0.407 | 27.53 ± 0.534 | 27.08 ± 0.46 |
| Fat-mass(kg) | 18.97 ± 0.249 | 18.64 ± 0.443 | 19.42 ± 0.589 | 18.90 ± 0.48 |
| LBM(kg) | 47.09 ± 0.222 | 46.93 ± 0.361 | 49.01 ± 0.506 | 48.90 ± 0.352 |
| **Muscle girth** | | | | |
| Forearm (cm) | 25.86 ± 0.07 | 25.71 ± 0.12 | 26.13 ± 0.16 | 25.71 ± 0.22 |
| Upperarm (cm) | 27.47 ± 0.11 | 27.19 ± 0.18 | 27.88 ± 0.22 | 27.57 ± 0.19 |
| Thigh (cm) | 50.16 ± 0.22 | 49.28 ± 0.36 | 50.0 ± 0.51 | 49.45 ± 0.40 |
| Calf (cm) | 35.09 ± 0.18 | 34.60 ± 0.24 | 35.08 ± 0.27 | 35.02 ± 0.21 |
| %MM | 25.81 ± 0.183 | 24.97 ± 0.251 | 25.12 ± 0.363 | 24.77 ± 0.308 |
| MM (kg) | 17.13 ± 0.176 | 16.48 ± 0.275 | 17.34 ± 0.387 | 16.91 ± 0.302 |

## Table 6. (Continued)

| Variables | Addictive Habits | | | |
|---|---|---|---|---|
| | Non-smoker Non-alcoholic (n = 594) | Smoker (n = 260) | Alcoholic (n = 148) | Smoker –Alcoholic (n = 214) |
| Bone width | | | | |
| Wrist* (cm) | 5.23 ± 0.01 | 5.19 ± 0.02 | 5.29 ± 0.03 | 5.28 ± 0.02 |
| Humerous* (cm) | 6.42 ± 0.02 | 6.43 ± 0.03 | 6.53 ± 0.04 | 6.53 ± 0.03 |
| Femur *(cm) | 9.29 ± 0.03 | 9.22 ± 0.04 | 9.41 ± 0.05 | 9.30 ± 0.04 |
| Ankle* (cm) | 6.78 ± 0.02 | 6.76 ± 0.03 | 6.89 ± 0.04 | 6.78 ± 0.03 |
| % SM | 11.43 ± 0.06 | 11.49 ± 0.108 | 11.50 ± 0.118 | 11.37 ± 0.108 |
| SM(kg) | 7.47 ± 0.044 | 7.41 ± 0.067 | 7.76 ± 0.091 | 7.61 ± 0.068 |
| Somatotype Component | | | | |
| Endomorphy | 5.09 ± 0.063 | 4.96 ± 0.107 | 4.94 ± 0.138 | 4.88 ± 0.118 |
| Mesomorphy | 4.02 ± 0.05 | 3.86 ± 0.088 | 4.09 ± 0.095 | 3.98 ± 0.094 |
| Ectomorphy | 2.06 ± 0.052 | 2.26 ± 0.097 | 2.04 ± 0.104 | 2.09 ± 0.091 |

Data were represented as Mean ± SE. * denotes statistical significance.

*Comparison of body composition and somatotype components among NS-NA, S, A and S-A:*

As noticed in Table 6, highest and lowest mean values of FM and LBM were found in the 'A' group and 'S' group, respectively. 'NS–NA' group had the highest %BF and lowest value of %BF was found among the 'S–A' group. So, it can be said that, 'A' group had more FM than any other group. %MM was highest among the 'NS–NA' group and lowest value was observed in 'S–A' group. MM was found to be highest among the A group and lowest in 'S' group. 'A'group also had highest %SM and SM when compared with other addictive habits. The mean somatotype of all the groups was found as mesomorphic endomorph. When compared among the different groups, highest endomorphy, mesomorphy and ectomorphy components were observed among 'NS–NA,' 'A' and 'S' group, respectively. Alcoholics were less ectomorphic, smokers were less mesomorphic and smoker-alcoholics were less endomorphic.

# DISCUSSION

## Smoking and Its Effects

Cigarette smoking is a major preventable cause of morbidity and mortality worldwide (Cokkinides et al., 2009). It is reported that >5 million people die worldwide from tobacco smoke-related illness each year (WHO, 2009). If this trend continues, it is expected that more than 08 million people will die annually from tobacco-related diseases by 2030 and more than 01 billion people during the 21st century (Shafey et al., 2009). In India, smoking is responsible for a large number of premature deaths affecting the prime working age group of 15–59 years (Jha et al., 2008). In the present study, it was observed that 39.1% people were addicted to smoking (Table 1) and light, moderate and heavy smoking was prevalent among 19.2%, 10.4% and 9.5% of the current smokers, respectively.

## Smoking and Cardiovascular System (CVS)

Inhaling tobacco smoke causes several immediate responses within the heart and its blood vessels (Cooney et al., 2010). The present study indicated elevated HR among the moderate and ex-smokers. It was also seen that heavy smokers had maximum SBP and DBP whereas both the values decreased for ex-smokers (Table 1). However, most of the cardiovascular diseases (CVD's) source is cigarette smoke which contain biologically active ingredients like nicotine, carbon monoxide (CO), oxidant gases and particulate matter (Brook and Rajagopalan, 2009). The probable mechanisms by which smoking increases HR and BP could be:

a. Mediated via direct stimulation of the sympathetic nervous system (Grassi et al., 1994).
b. The main addictive substance in cigarettes, nicotine, stimulates the body to produce adrenaline which causes subsequent increase in content of plasma adrenalin and makes the heart beat faster and also increases BP (Primatesta et al., 2001).
c. Smoking increases CO levels in blood and produces carboxyhemoglobins which makes the tissue starved for oxygenated blood, cause them to suffocate and die, making smokers to experience shortness of breath and increased HR.
d. Another major contribution to the increased risk of CVD among smokers is tobacco's effect on increasing overall blood cholesterol levels. This may be due to presence of acrolein which affects the way the body processes cholesterol, allowing greater amounts to remain in the blood system, causing sudden blockage of an artery, leading to a fatal heart attack and stroke (Tamamizu-Kato et al., 2007).
e. Smoking causes the body's blood vessels to constrict (vasoconstriction) by decreasing nitrous oxide (NO), resulting in raising BP (Kiowski et al., 1994).

Similar to other reports, our study also showed higher prevalence of HTN among heavy smokers (Figure 2) which could be due to vascular endothelium dysfunction (Panwar et al., 2011; Talukder et al., 2010; Jatoi et al., 2007). The precise mechanisms of cigarette smoking-induced endothelium dysfunction are not fully understood, but several potential mechanisms are likely to be involved.

a. Oxidative damage seems to constitute the primary mechanism because cigarette smoking contains a large number of oxidants and introduces reactive oxygen species (ROS) in the circulatory system (Csiszar et al., 2009).
b. ROS generated by long-term smoking may directly damage endothelial cells and inactivate NO (Csiszar et al., 2009).
c. Decreased NO release, dysfunctional NO synthase and increased NO consumption, are linked with endothelium dysfunction in healthy smokers (Csiszar et al., 2009).

Moreover, decreased physical activity and increased alcohol consumption (Figure 1) was also found higher among the current smokers which may contribute to increased prevalence of HTN, under study. Similar results with peculiar lifestyle pattern were also reported by other studies where smokers drink more alcohol and engage in less physical activity (Ahmed & Memon, 2008; Chiolero et al., 2006).

## Smoking and Obesity

According to the Framingham study, the life expectancy of obese smokers was 13 years less than that of normal-weight nonsmokers (Peeters et al., 2003). Numerous cross-sectional studies indicate that cigarette smoking has an inverse association with body weight or body mass index (BMI; in $kg/m^2$) (Canoy et al., 2005; Huot et al., 2004). In the present study, a similar result was observed where current smokers had lower BMI and they also weighed less than non-smokers and ex-smokers (Table 1). It was also observed from Figure 2 that the proportion of obese individuals was higher for non-smokers compared to current smokers. Smoking's effect could lead to loss in body weight by decreasing metabolic efficiency or reducing caloric absorption (reduction in appetite). This metabolic effect of smoking could explain the lower body weight found in smokers (Chiolero et al., 2008). Besides its metabolic properties, increasing doses of nicotine could induce an acute anorexic effect which reduces hunger and food consumption and increases the feeling of fullness (Jessen et al., 2005), and as a result body weight decreased. Available reports have indicated that current smokers are less likely to be physically active (Chiolero et al., 2006) and habituated to irregular dietary pattern (Kaczynski et al., 2008). This was also supported by our finding where the majority of the smokers were alcohol consumers and physically inactive (Figure 1).

There is increasing evidence which have examined the relationship between smoking and body shape and reported that smoking is associated with central obesity (Chhabra & Chhabra, 2011; Houston et al., 2006). Cross-sectional studies indicate that smokers tend to have a larger WC and WHR than nonsmokers and they also had greater abdominal obesity (Chhabra & Chhabra, 2011; Leite & Nicolosi, 2006); these findings reflect greater abdominal fat deposition. The present study is a contradiction from the above-mentioned results, where it was found that the current smokers had lower WC, and similar WHR and WHtR than non-smokers (Table 1). Most of the reports showed that heavy smokers (>20 cigarettes/day) have greater body weight and increased obesity than light smokers (1-9 cigarettes/day) (Chiolero et al., 2007; John et al., 2005). However, in the present study, smokers were found mostly either light or moderate and only a few of them were heavy smokers. Probably this may be the reason why smokers in this study had lower mean values of obesity indices and lower prevalence of obesity among them.

In line with other studies (Bush et al., 2016; Aubin et al., 2012), it has been reflected in our study too that smoking cessation causes weight gain, increases the mean values of obesity parameters (Table 1), and prevalence of overall, abdominal and truncal obesity (Figure 2). Smokers gain weight after they quit smoking primarily because of the removal of nicotine's effects on the central nervous system. Some smokers also attempt to cope with nicotine withdrawal by substituting eating for the 'hand to mouth' behavior of smoking which can lead to an increase in caloric intake. Moreover, low satiety, emotional eating, calorie misperception and short sleep might also contribute to post cessation weight gain (Biedermann et al., 2013; Komiyama et al., 2013). It has also been suggested that, in many people, the sudden drop in blood sugar during the first three days of quitting smoking could lead to common withdrawal symptoms such as headaches, dizziness and craving for sweets (Rodin, 1987) which, in turn, could lead to overeating in an attempt to cope with these symptoms (Komiyama et al., 2013).

## Smoking and DM

It was reported that the risk of Type II DM is greater in current smokers than nonsmokers (Akter et al., 2017; Pan et al., 2015). The result of our study also corroborates with the above mentioned finding where current smokers showed higher mean value of RBS and higher prevalence of DM (Table 1 and Figure 2). The association between smoking and Type II DM is biologically plausible and the probable reasons are as follows:

a. Smoking leads to insulin resistance or inadequate insulin secretion due to oxidative stress, inflammation and endothelial dysfunction (Yanbaeva et al., 2007).
b. Nicotine in cigarette can cause β-cell dysfunction, increase β-cell apoptosis and loss of β-cell mass (Bruin et al., 2008).
c. In addition, although smoking tends to decrease body weight, it leads to central adiposity, which has been linked to inflammation and insulin resistance (Chhabra & Chhabra, 2011; Bastard et al., 2006; Kahn et al., 2006).

Apart from this, increased alcohol consumption and lower physical activity, increased prevalence of family history of DM may be the basis of increased DM among the current smokers.

It was observed that ex-smokers had higher mean values of RBS and higher prevalence of DM (Table 1 & Figure 2) compared to non-smokers and current smokers. The results obtained under study is comparable with the literature where quitting tobacco seems to worsen glycemic control and increase the risk for new onset of Type II DM (Akter et al., 2017; Bush et al., 2016). The mechanism by which tobacco cessation leads to DM onset or poorer DM control is not clear but the increased risk was explained by several researchers are as follows (Bush et al., 2016; Stadler et al., 2014; Perkins et al., 1990):

a. Increases in visceral fat accumulation or excessive weight gain after quitting smoking.
b. Deterioration of insulin sensitivity and lipid profiles after smoking cessation.
c. Greater consumption of sugary foods and carbohydrates.

## Alcohol and Its Effects

The burden of alcohol use poses a serious threat to human civilization. Globally, harmful use of alcohol causes approximately 3.3 million deaths every year and 5.1% global burden of disease is attributable to alcohol consumption (WHO, 2016). Lim et al., (2012) found that alcohol was the third leading risk factor for death and disability. Overall, alcohol consumption is estimated to account for 5% of all cancer deaths worldwide and it is significant in low and middle-income countries (Weiderpass, 2010). Despite the growing global interest in the alcohol related problem, fewer reports are available about the prevalence of alcohol use in many developing countries. In an alarming revelation, WHO (2016) states that the amount of alcohol consumption has risen in India between the periods 2008 to 2012. In India, alcohol consumption is one of the risk factors and attributable to nearly 3% of disability-adjusted life years lost (Lim et al., 2012). Finally, alcohol consumption has been identified as a cause for more than 200 diseases, injuries and other health conditions (Rehm et al., 2010).

Large or nationally representative studies on alcohol consumption have not been conducted in India due to resource constraints. A limited number of studies have been conducted on smaller groups in different regions of India. Rajeev et al., (2017) studied on rural people of Kerala in India and reported 12.6% prevalence of habitual drinking. Pati et al., (2017) reported 38% prevalence of alcohol consumption and of those 60% was hazardous drinkers. Reports were also available on the people of Andaman and Nicobar Islands and it was found that 20.7% of the people were addicted to alcohol (Manimunda et al., 2017). In the present study, prevalence of current alcohol consumption was 30.1% (Table 2) which is higher than the prevalence reported by Manimunda et al., (2017) and Rajeev et al., (2017) and lower than a study conducted by Pati et al., (2017).

## Alcohol Consumption and CVS

The present study observed significantly increased HR, SBP and DBP values among the current alcoholics and the mean values of these variables increased with the amount of alcohol consumption (Table 2). Slagter et al., (2014) and Taylor et al., (2009) also reported similar finding on alcohol consumption. The results obtained from our study showed increased prevalence of HTN among the current alcoholics. In comparison to non-alcoholics, 35%, 50% and 53% of the light, moderate and heavy drinkers, respectively, were hypertensive (Figure 4). In corroboration to the present study, other studies also showed that people consuming more alcohol had a higher risk of developing HTN (Venkataraman et al., 2013; Sumeet et al., 2011). Even one drink in a day can increase the HTN risk and the overall risk climbs higher for every drink after that. The relationship remains significant even when age, gender, ethnicity, diet, exercise and smoking habits are taken into account (Briasoulis et al., 2012; Taylor et al., 2009).

So, it can be said that alcohol consumption is one of the most controllable and preventable risk factors for HTN. Different research groups suggested several possible mechanisms through which alcohol can raise BP, as follows:

a. Alcohol increases sympathetic nervous system activity that constricts blood vessels and increases the contractile force of the heart (Russ et al., 1991).
b. Alcohol decreases sensitivity of baroreceptors in the artery walls, reducing signals to the central nervous system that are required to normalize BP (el-Mas & Abdel-Rahman, 1993).
c. Certain studies have implicated the role of cortisol in alcohol-induced rise in BP. Potter et al., (1986) has reported a significant rise in plasma cortisol levels following alcohol consumption which may be due to direct stimulation of adreno-corticotropin hormone or potentiation of corticotropin releasing hormones by arginine vasopressin. The effect on BP may also be due to the mineralocorticoid activity of cortisol or catecholamine hypersensitivity (Bannan et al., 1984).
d. The mechanisms of alcohol-mediated HTN also include potentiation of the renin-angiotensin-aldosterone system (RAAS). This is reflected in significantly elevated circulating angiotensin II levels (Cheng et al., 2006), elevated cardiac angiotensin converting enzyme expression (Kim et al., 2001) and increased cardiac expression of angiotensin type 1 receptors (AT1R) (Cheng et al., 2006). AT1R have been associated with ventricular dysfunction, elevations of end-diastolic pressure, and alcohol-induced vascular injury (Cheng et al., 2006).
e. Vasdev et al., (1991) have shown that increases in cytosolic free calcium and calcium uptake are associated with alcohol induced HTN. It was proposed that alcohol increases intracellular $Ca^{2+}$ by (a) direct up regulation of voltage-gated $Ca^{2+}$ channels; (b) inhibition of $Ca^{2+}$-adenosine triphosphatase ($Ca^{2+}$-ATPase) that extrudes $Ca^{2+}$ from the cells; and (c) magnesium ion ($Mg^{2+}$)

depletion that inhibits the sodium ion ($Na^+$)-potassium ion ($K^+$) pump ($Na^+/K^+$-ATPase), causing a buildup of intracellular $Na^+$. This reaction in turn inhibits the $Na^+/ Ca^{2+}$ exchanger, thereby increasing the intracellular calcium ion. Finally, alcohol reduces the ratio of ionized Mg to ionized Ca in plasma, resulting in an increase in BP as the vessels contract (Altura & Altura, 1994).

Moreover, increased SLT consumption, smoking habits, sedentary lifestyle and increased family history of HTN among the alcoholics (Figure 3) may also contribute to the increased cardiovascular parameters and HTN prevalence.

## Alcohol Consumption and Obesity

Alcohol consumption is correlated with increased risk for overall body obesity (Lukasiewicz et al., 2005) as well as abdominal obesity (Lourenco et al., 2012; Ryu et al., 2010). Similar to a study done by Slagter et al., (2014), we also found that the individuals who consumed alcohol had a higher BMI, WC, WHR and WHtR and obesity prevalence (Table 2 & Figure 4). The probable mechanisms for alcoholic obesity have been suggested in various studies which include:

a. Release of the neurotransmitter dopamine, a component of the brain's reward system, is stimulated by alcohol intake (Trinko et al., 2007) and also plays a role in the rewarding properties of eating and overeating (Wang et al., 2001). Alcohol acts on the opioid neurotransmitter system which is also associated with the regulation of the sensory reward components of eating (Yeomans & Gray, 2002). Finally, alcohol binds to opioid, serotonergic and gamma aminobutyric acid (GABA) receptors that have been implicated in the motivation to drink more alcohol (Lobo & Harris, 2008).

b. Alcohol influences taste or stimulates appetite and increases hunger (Yeomans, 2010). Alternatively, alcohol may increase energy intake by interfering with mechanisms of satiety or "fullness" (Breslow et al., 2013; Caton et al., 2005) and inhibiting the effects of leptin or glucagon-like peptide-1 (GLP-1) (Röjdmark et al., 2001).
c. Alcohol inhibits fat oxidation, suggesting that frequent alcohol consumption could lead to fat sparing, and thus higher BF in the long term (Lukasiewicz et al., 2005).
d. Alcohol may contribute to abdominal obesity through non-caloric mechanisms such as, alterations of steroid hormones that favor central fat storage (Björntorp, 1995), increased cortisol secretion (Kissebah & Krakower, 1994) and a lower secretion of lipid mobilizing sex steroid hormones which promotes visceral fat accumulation (Björntorp, 1995).
e. Alcohol intake may be associated with altered patterns of nutrient intake (Thomson et al., 1988), resulting in the substitution of alcohol for other nutrients.
f. According to Suter &Tremblay (2005), other factors may also influence the relationship between alcohol intake and body weight, including the frequency of drinking, gender, genetic background and diet.

## Alcohol Consumption and DM

A dual relationship exists between alcohol consumption and risk of DM where light or moderate drinking may be beneficial and heavy drinking is detrimental (Baliunas et al., 2009; Carlsson et al., 2005). In the comparative study among the different categories of alcoholics, the RBS value was found significantly higher among the current drinkers, especially among the light drinkers (Table 2). Koppes et al., (2005) and Carlsson et al., (2005) reported that alcohol consumption is associated with decreased occurrence of DM. Similar results were also obtained in our study showing lower prevalence of DM among the current drinkers (except light drinkers) and the data was represented in Figure 4. The possible reasons could be an increase in HDL cholesterol (Rimm et al., 1999) and the anti-inflammatory effect of alcohol (Hendriks, 2007).

Available literature indicates that moderate alcohol consumption is associated with decreased risk of Type II DM (Zhang et al., 2016; Schrieks et al., 2015). Our study also observed lower mean RBS value and DM prevalence among the moderate drinkers (Table 2 & Figure 4). This beneficial effect of moderate alcohol consumption on risk of Type II DM could be explained by the enhanced insulin sensitivity due to long term intake of moderate amount of alcohol (Koppes et al., 2005; Van de Wiel, 2004).

## Combined Effects of Smoking and Alcohol

It's no mystery that smoking and drinking go hand in hand. So far, we have considered the effects of smoking and drinking as separate behaviors but in fact they often occur together. Pati et al., (2017) reported that smokers were eight times more likely to be alcoholics and the prevalence of alcohol drinking was four times higher in tobacco users. Pharmacologically, ethanol and nicotine have counteracting effects which partially titrate each other. Lĕ et al., (2000) said that repeated administrations of nicotine stimulate alcohol consumption whereas Johnson et al., (1991) and Chen et al., (2001) proposed that nicotine reduces the intoxicating effects of alcohol. As the desired effect of alcohol is significantly diminished by nicotine, cigarette smoking appears to promote the consumption of alcohol. Some of the other studies have examined the combined effects of smoking and drinking on mortality. Premature mortality was particularly high in smokers who drank ≥15 units/day, 25% of the population were not surviving to age 65 years (Hart et al., 2010).

Alcohol and smoking have opposite effects on insulin sensitivity, with alcohol having favorable effects (Koppes et al., 2005). A further contrast was also observed in between these two factors on the effect of BP. Alcohol consumption of ≥ 3 drinks/day increases BP (Taylor et al., 2009) whereas the relationship between smoking and BP is less clear or even non-existent (Slagter et al., 2013; Narkiewicz et al., 2005). The results obtained in the present study depicted a progressive increase in the percentage of pre-hypertension (pre-HTN) and HTN with concomitant use of both alcohol and smoking (Table 3). However, both smoking and alcohol consumption seem to have a positive association with abdominal obesity which is supported by our study observation (Table 3) and also other groups (Slagter et al., 2013; Saarni et al, 2009). It was seen that the prevalence of obesity also increased for both alcoholics and smoker-alcoholics cases. Finally, it can be said that the Alcoholic group ('A' group) was in the risk zone for developing obesity and HTN whereas Smoker-Alcoholic group ('S-A' group) had the risk to get DM.

## Addictive Habits, Body Composition and Somatotype

### *Effect of Alcohol and Smoking on FM*

**Alcohol Consumption**

Drinking alcoholic beverages is a common feature of social gatherings. Aside from fat, ethanol is a macronutrient with high energy density and it affects the individual's total daily energy intake. There is a paradoxical relationship between the amount of alcohol consumption and body weight for chronic/heavy alcohol drinkers. In fact, weight loss, temporal fat loss, peculiar body composition and malnutrition are commonly observed in chronic drinkers (Addolorato et al., 2000). Table 5 shows that, biceps, triceps, suprailiac SKFs and %BF was increased among light and heavy drinkers but lowered for moderate drinkers. Moreover, Subscapular and mid-thigh SKFs was decreased with an increase in drinking frequency. Abdominal SKF, FM and LBM values showed a linear increasing pattern with the amount of alcohol consumption and the possible mechanisms are as follows:

a. Alcohol influences taste or stimulates appetite and increases hunger. As a result, overall energy intake is often increased following alcohol consumption (Breslow et al., 2013; Yeomans, 2010).
b. Alcohol may also increase energy intake by interfering with mechanisms of satiety or "fullness." (Caton et al. 2005).
c. Apart from the immediate influence on appetite, alcohol also increases energy storage. Alcohol inhibits fat oxidation and encourages further alcohol intake, resulting in higher BF for long term (Lukasiewicz et al., 2005).

**Smoking**

Table 4 represents that among the current smokers, thickness of all the SKFs, %BF and FM decreases in a liner fashion with increase in number of cigarettes smoked/day. The main ingredient of tobacco is nicotine which decreases metabolic efficiency and calorie absorption, resulting in reduced FM and %BF among the smokers and SLT users. Moreover, nicotine could encourage an acute anorexic effect which reduces food consumption and increases the feeling of fullness (Jessen et al., 2005; Chiolero et al., 2008).

**Combined Effect of Smoking and Alcohol**

In the present investigation, Table 6 shows that 'A' group had highest mean values of FM and LBM which could be due to higher energy intake through alcohol's effect on appetite stimulation. Long term alcohol consumption also affects energy storage by inhibiting fat oxidation leading to fat sparing and increased FM. It was also revealed that smoker group (S group) had lowest FM and LBM (Table 6). The presence of nicotine in tobacco encourages acute anorexic effect and reduces food consumption which decreases metabolic efficiency and calorie absorption. Table 6 also indicated that 'S-A' group had lower FM than non-smoker non-alcoholic group (NS-NA group) and 'A' group, but higher than the 'S' group. The decrease of FM in 'S-A' group could be due to the effect of active ingredient of tobacco (nicotine).

## Effect of Alcohol and Smoking on MM

### Alcohol Consumption

Most of the reports said that chronic alcohol ingestion reduces protein synthesis and decreases MM. In the present study, an interesting observation was shown that current alcoholics had little increment in mean values of all the muscle girths and MM compare to non-alcoholic counterparts (Table 5). Therefore, it may be said that alcohol consumption had insignificant effects on skeletal muscle and protein synthesis, in our study area.

### Smoking

A Linear decreasing trend was observed for all muscle girths, %MM and MM among the smokers (Table 4). It was seen that smoking affects MM by decreasing the rate of muscle renewal and depressed muscle protein synthesis (Rennie et al., 2004). The reduction of muscle protein synthesis may be due to the direct effect of nicotine or an indirect effect of life style, more specifically alcohol consumption and physical activity attitudes among smokers.

### Combined Effect of Smoking and Alcohol

The effect of both smoking and alcohol on MM was shown in Table 6. It was seen that the 'A' group had highest MM which contradicts with previous study (Vary and Lang, 2008). Furthermore, Table 6 was also indicated that 'S' group had lowest MM. This might be due to a direct effect of nicotine which reduces muscle protein synthesis (Rennie et al., 2004). However, the observed results of MM for both smoker and alcoholics were in between 'S' and 'A' group and the MM follows the order as 'S'< 'S-A'< 'A'.

## Effect of Alcohol and Smoking on Bone Health

**Alcohol Consumption**

Table 5 shows increased bone widths and SM among the current alcoholics and similar observation was also made by Díez et al., (1994). The background reasons for increasing bone density with alcohol consumption have not yet been established, but proposed mechanisms for this positive association include:

- a. A reduction in bone remodeling via decrease in parathyroid hormone concentrations and an increase in calcitonin production (a hormone involved in the metabolism of bone) (Jugdaohsingh et al., 2006);
- b. Increased production of adrenal androstenedione which sequentially converts to estrogen. The increased estrogen may increase bone density (Kim et al., 2003);
- c. The high silicon content of beer and the phenolic constituents of alcoholic beverages may promote bone formation (Jugdaohsingh et al., 2006).

On the other hand, present study also indicated reduced %SM among the current drinkers (Table 5). The mechanism for this association is not clearly understood, however, some potential factors include (Ilich & Kerstetter, 2000):

- a. Poor nutrition and mal absorption of nutrients;
- b. Alterations in the metabolism of vitamin D and calcium;
- c. Potential toxic effects of excessive alcohol intake on osteoblasts, thus impairing their function.

**Smoking**

It was found that all the bone widths and SM decreased among the heavy smokers compared to non-smokers (Table 4). Smoking reduces bone density in various ways, like

a. Smoking decreases estrogen levels and reduces calcium absorption by decreasing parathyroid hormone whereas cortisol and adrenal androgen level increases. These hormonal changes lead to lower bone density (Kapoor & Jones, 2005).
b. Smoking reduces the level of Vitamin D in the body which is required for good bone health (Brot et al., 1999);
c. Smoking increases free radicals and oxidative stress which affects bone reabsorption (Duthie et al., 1991).
d. Smokers are more likely to suffer from peripheral vascular disease hence reducing blood supply to the bones (Vestergaard & Mosekilde, 2003).
e. Smoking also adversely affects other hormones and enzymes involved in bone regulation, including parathyroid hormone and alkaline phosphatase (Landin-Wilhelmsen et al., 1995; Gordon, 1993).
f. Finally, direct toxic effects of many constituents of tobacco may affect bone cells (Broulik & Jarab, 1993).

Slight increment in some bone widths, %SM and SM among the light and moderate smokers (Table 4) was observed which may be due to their engagement in leisure time physical activity. It was also noted that smoking cessation showed a beneficial role on bone mass by increasing bone widths, %SM and SM.

**Combined Effect of Smoking and Alcohol**

It was noticeable that 'A' group had highest %SM and SM which might be due to decrease in parathyroid hormone concentration and increase in calcitonin production. These two hormones reduce bone remodeling and increase bone metabolism, respectively. Moreover, increased production of estrogen may also increase bone density among alcoholics only. Table 6 indicates that the 'S' group had the lowest mean value of SM, due to tobacco's effect. Smoking reduces the level of Vitamin D and increases free radicals and oxidative stress in the body which affects bone reabsorption and SM decreases. Tobacco and alcohol produce some negative and positive effect on SM, respectively, due to which 'S-A' group had lower SM than 'A' group and higher SM than 'S' group.

## *Effect of Alcohol and Smoking on Somatotype*

### Alcohol Consumption

In the present study, all alcoholics were observed as mesomorphic-endomorph (Table 5). Compared to non-drinkers, endomorphy rating decreased among current drinkers which could be due to decreased %BF. Among the current alcoholics, light drinkers have improved MM for an increase in mesomorphy rating. Ectomorphy rating decreased among light and heavy drinkers, whereas moderate drinkers were more ectomorphic.

### Smoking

Endomorphy and mesomorphy ratings showed a linear declining trend with rising smoking pattern whereas ectomorphy rating followed reverse trend (Table 4). Nicotine was the main responsible component for decreasing both endomorphy (reduced calorie absorption and induced anorexic effect) and mesomorphy rating (higher loss in MM) (Chiolero et al., 2008; Jessen et al., 2005; Rennie et al., 2004).

### Combined Effect of Smoking and Alcohol

The mean somatotype of all the groups was observed from Table 6, as mesomorphic-endomorph. Highest endomorphy, mesomorphy and ectomorphy components were seen among 'NS-NA' group, 'A' group and 'S' group, respectively. So, it can be said that alcoholics were less ectomorphic, smokers were less mesomorphic whereas smoker-alcoholics were less endomorphic.

# CONCLUSION

The findings of this study reveal that a notable number of Kolkata based people are addicted to alcohol consumption and smoking. These addictions increased the prevalence of obese, hypertensive and diabetic people. Changes in several body compositions and somatotype parameters were also observed due to the changes in lifestyle. Further in-depth research is recommended to identify the other associated lifestyle and environmental factors which might be involved in producing these conditions. Lifestyle modifications should be used as initial therapy to control the increasing prevalence of lifestyle induced diseases.

In conclusion, the present study highlights major issues that should be dealt with both at primary health care level and at a community level. Considering the high prevalence of NCD risk factors and NCDs, the effect of prevention may be substantial. Associations between several lifestyle factors like smoking, alcohol consumption and NCDs, further emphasize the need of focusing on lifestyle modifications to prevent further development of concerned NCDs. Last but not the least, it is to be mentioned that though there are acts framed by the Government of India prohibiting cigarette smoking and other tobacco products at public places including bars and restaurants (Cigarettes and Other Tobacco Products (Prohibition of Advertisement and Regulation of Trade and Commerce, Production, Supply and Distribution) Act, 2003, COTPA, 2003), proper implementation and surveillance by the competent authorities of different states should be ensured. Similar act also exists in the state of West Bengal entitled "The West Bengal Prohibition of Smoking and Spitting and Protection of Health of Non-smokers and Minors Act, 2001," however, proper enforcement of the act should be ascertained.

## Socio-Physiological Implication

- This cross-sectional study on Kolkata based people may provide a databank regarding lifestyle pattern induced physiological changes and prevalence of lifestyle induced NCDs and Government of West Bengal will not have to depend on other agencies.
- These data can be used for comparison if further investigations are to be carried out in the relevant field in future.

- Identified risk factors associated with mode of lifestyle might provide important clues to the Health Care Providers in improving adult addiction cessation counseling program for addictives.
- Different health Insurance companies may use these data to formulate their own policies for different age groups depending on the risk factor associated with lifestyle pattern particularly for younger age group.
- These data may also be utilized in campaigns organized by different Government and Non-Government Organizations as well as in Community Health Programs to educate and aware people of their general health.
- These data may serve to propel multi-sectoral efforts to lower the community burden of NCD risk factors in India in general, and in Kolkata, in particular.

## Acknowledgments

The authority of Rammohan College is greatly acknowledged for providing infrastructural facilities to carry out this research. The individuals who participated in the study are also deeply acknowledged.

## References

Addolorato, G., Capristo, E., Marini, M., Santini, P., Scognamiglio, U., Attilia, M. L., and Ceccanti, M. (2000). Body composition changes induced by chronic ethanol abuse: evaluation by dual energy X-ray absorptiometry. *The American Journal of Gastroenterology*, 95 (9): 2323-2327. doi:10.1111/j.1572-0241.2000.02320.x.

Ahmed, S. T., and Memon, M. A. (2008). Smoking and its relationship with blood pressure, blood glucose and blood parameters in patients with coronary heart disease. *Pakistan Journal of Physiology*, 4 (1): 5-7. doi: http://www.pjp.pps.org.pk/index.php/PJP/article/view/638.

Akter, S., Goto, A., and Mizoue, T. (2017). Smoking and the risk of type 2 diabetes in Japan: A systematic review and meta-analysis. *Journal of Epidemiology*, 27 (12): 553-561. doi: 10.1016/j.je.2016.12.017.

Altura, B. M., and Altura, B. T. (1994). Role of magnesium and calcium in alcohol-induced hypertension and strokes as probed by In Vivo Television Microscopy, Digital Image Microscopy, Optical Spectroscopy, 31P-NMR, Spectroscopy and a unique Magnesium Ion-Selective Electrode. *Alcoholism: Clinical and Experimental Research*, 18 (5): 1057-1068. doi: 10.1111/j.1530-0277.1994.tb00082.x.

American Diabetes Association. (2016). 2. Classification and diagnosis of diabetes. *Diabetes Care*, 39 (Supplement 1), S13-S22. doi: https://doi.org/10.2337/DC16-S005.

Ashwell, M., and Gibson, S. (2016). Waist-to-height ratio as an indicator of 'early health risk': simpler and more predictive than using a 'matrix' based on BMI and waist circumference. *BMJ Open*, 6 (3): e010159. doi: http://dx.doi.org/10.1136/bmjopen-2015-010159.

Aubin, H. J., Farley, A., Lycett, D., Lahmek, P., and Aveyard, P. (2012). Weight gain in smokers after quitting cigarettes: meta-analysis. *BMJ*, 345: e4439. doi: https://doi.org/10.1136/bmj.e4439.

Baliunas, D. O., Taylor, B. J., Irving, H., Roerecke, M., Patra, J., Mohapatra, S., and Rehm, J. (2009). Alcohol as a risk factor for type 2 diabetes: a systematic review and meta-analysis. *Diabetes Care*, 32 (11): 2123-2132. doi: 10.2337/dc09-0227.

Bannan, L. T., Potter, J. F., Beevers, D. G., Saunders, J. B., Walters, J. R. F., and Ingram, M. C. (1984). Effect of alcohol withdrawal on blood pressure, plasma renin activity, aldosterone, cortisol and dopamine β-hydroxylase. *Clinical Science*, 66 (6): 659-663. doi: 10.1042/cs0660659.

Bastard, J. P., Maachi, M., Lagathu, C., Kim, M. J., Caron, M., Vidal, H., and Feve, B. (2006). Recent advances in the relationship between obesity, inflammation, and insulin resistance. *European Cytokine*

*Network,* 17 (1): 4-12. https://www.ncbi.nlm.nih.gov/pubmed/16613757.

Biedermann, L., Zeitz, J., Mwinyi, J., Sutter-Minder, E., Rehman, A., Ott, S. J. and Loessner, M. J. (2013). Smoking cessation induces profound changes in the composition of the intestinal microbiota in humans. *PloS one*, 8 (3): e59260. doi: 10.1371/journal.pone.0059260.

Björntorp, P. (1995). Endocrine abnormalities of obesity. *Metabolism-Clinical and Experimental*, 44: 21-23. doi: 10.1016/0026-0495(95)90315-1.

Breslow, R. A., Chen, C. M., Graubard, B. I., Jacobovits, T., and Kant, A. K. (2013). Diets of drinkers on drinking and nondrinking days: NHANES 2003–2008. *The American Journal of Clinical Nutrition*, 97 (5): 1068-1075. doi: 10.3945/ajcn.112.050161.

Briasoulis, A., Agarwal, V., and Messerli, F. H. (2012). Alcohol consumption and the risk of hypertension in men and women: a systematic review and meta-analysis. *The Journal of Clinical Hypertension*, 14 (11): 792-798. doi: 10.1111/jch.12008.

Brook, R. D., and Rajagopalan, S. (2009). Particulate matter, air pollution, and blood pressure. *Journal of the American Society of Hypertension*, 3 (5): 332-350. doi: 10.1016/j.jash.2009.08.005.

Brot, C., Jorgensen, N. R., and Sorensen, O. H. (1999). The influence of smoking on vitamin D status and calcium metabolism. *European Journal of Clinical Nutrition*, 53 (12): 920–926. doi: 10.1038/sj.ejcn.1600870.

Broulik, P. D., and Jarab, J. (1993). The effect of chronic nicotine administration on bone mineral content in mice. *Hormone and Metabolic Research*, 25 (4): 219–221. doi: 10.1055/s-2007-1002080.

Bruin, J. E., Gerstein, H. C., Morrison, K. M., and Holloway, A. C. (2008). Increased pancreatic beta-cell apoptosis following fetal and neonatal exposure to nicotine is mediated via the mitochondria. *Toxicological Sciences*, 103 (2): 362-370. doi: 10.1093/toxsci/kfn012.

Bush, T., Lovejoy, J. C., Deprey, M., and Carpenter, K. M. (2016). The effect of tobacco cessation on weight gain, obesity, and diabetes risk. *Obesity*, 24 (9): 1834-1841. doi: 10.1002/oby.21582.

Canoy, D., Wareham, N., Luben, R., Welch, A., Bingham, S., Day, N., and Khaw, K. T. (2005). Cigarette smoking and fat distribution in 21, 828 British men and women: a population-based study. *Obesity*, 13 (8): 1466-1475. doi: 10.1038/oby.2005.177.

Carlsson, S., Hammar, N., and Grill, V. (2005). Alcohol consumption and type 2 diabetes. *Diabetologia*, 48 (6): 1051-1054. doi: 10.1007/s00125-005-1768-5.

Carter, J. L., and Heath, B. H. (1990). *Somatotyping: development and applications* (Vol. 5). New York: Cambridge University Press.

Caton, S. J., Marks, J. E., and Hetherington, M. M. (2005). Pleasure and alcohol: manipulating pleasantness and the acute effects of alcohol on food intake. *Physiology & Behavior*, 84 (3): 371-377. doi: https://doi.org/10.1016/j.physbeh.2004.12.013.

Chakma, J. K., and Gupta, S. (2014). Lifestyle and non-communicable diseases: A double edged sword for future India. *Indian Journal of Community Health*, 26 (4): 325-332. https://www.iapsmupuk.org/journal/index.php/IJCH/article/view/434.

Chen, W. J. A., Parnell, S. E., and West, J. R. (2001). Nicotine decreases blood alcohol concentration in neonatal rats. *Alcoholism: Clinical and Experimental Research*, 25 (7): 1072-1077. doi: https://doi.org/10.1111/j.1530-0277.2001.tb02319.x.

Cheng, C. P., Cheng, H. J., Cunningham, C., Shihabi, Z. K., Sane, D. C., Wannenburg, T., and Little, W. C. (2006). Angiotensin II type 1 receptor blockade prevents alcoholic cardiomyopathy. *Circulation*, 114 (3): 226-236. doi: 10.1161/CIRCULATIONAHA.105.596494.

Chhabra, P., & Chhabra, S. K. (2011). Effect of smoking on body mass index: a community-based study. *National Journal of Community Medicine*, 2 (3): 325-330.

Chiolero, A., Faeh, D., Paccaud, F., and Cornuz, J. (2008). Consequences of smoking for body weight, body fat distribution, and insulin resistance. *The American Journal of Clinical Nutrition*, 87 (4): 801-809. doi: 10.1093/ajcn/87.4.801.

Chiolero, A., Jacot-Sadowski, I., Faeh, D., Paccaud, F., and Cornuz, J. (2007). Association of cigarettes smoked daily with obesity in a general adult population. *Obesity*, 15 (5): 1311-1318. doi: 10.1038/oby.2007.153.

Chiolero, A., Wietlisbach, V., Ruffieux, C., Paccaud, F., & Cornuz, J. (2006). Clustering of risk behaviors with cigarette consumption: a population-based survey. *Preventive Medicine*, 42 (5): 348-353. doi: 10.1016/j.ypmed.2006.01.011.

Cokkinides, V., Bandi, P., McMahon, C., Jemal, A., Glynn, T., and Ward, E. (2009). Tobacco control in the United States—recent progress and opportunities. *CA: A Cancer Journal for Clinicians*, 59 (6): 352-365. doi: 10.3322/caac.20037.

Cooney, M. T., Vartiainen, E., Laakitainen, T., Juolevi, A., Dudina, A., and Graham, I. M. (2010). Elevated resting heart rate is an independent risk factor for cardiovascular disease in healthy men and women. *American Heart Journal*, 159 (4): 612-619. doi: 10.1016/j.ahj.2009.12.029.

Csiszar, A., Podlutsky, A., Wolin, M. S., Losonczy, G., Pacher, P., and Ungvari, Z. (2009). Oxidative stress and accelerated vascular aging: implications for cigarette smoking. *Frontiers in Bioscience: A Journal and Virtual Library*, 14: 3128-3144. doi: https://doi.org/10.2741/3440.

Díez, A., Puig, J., Serrano, S., Marinoso, M. L., Bosch, J., Marrugat, J., and Aubía, J. (1994). Alcohol-induced bone disease in the absence of severe chronic liver damage. *Journal of Bone and Mineral Research*, 9 (6): 825-831. doi: https://doi.org/10.1002/jbmr.5650090608.

Drinkwater, D. T., Martin, A. D., Ross, W. D., and Clarys, J. P. (1986). Validation by cadaver dissection of Matiegka's equations for the anthropometric estimation of anatomical body composition in adult humans. In *the 1984 Olympic Scientific Congress Proceedings: Perspectives in Kinanthropometry (Ed. JA Day) Human Kinetics, Champaign* (Vol. 221, p. 227).

Durnin, J. V., and Womersley, J. V. G. A. (1974). Body fat assessed from total body density and its estimation from skinfold thickness: measurements on 481 men and women aged from 16 to 72 years. *British Journal of Nutrition*, 32 (1): 77-97. doi: https://doi.org/10.1079/BJN19740060.

Duthie, G. G., Arthur, J. R., and James, W. P. T. (1991). Effects of smoking and vitamin E on blood antioxidant status. *The American Journal of Clinical Nutrition*, 53 (4): 1061S-1063S. doi: https://doi.org/10.1093/ajcn/53.4.1061S.

el-Mas, M. M., and Abdel-Rahman, A. A. (1993). Direct evidence for selective involvement of aortic baroreceptors in ethanol-induced impairment of baroreflex control of heart rate. *Journal of Pharmacology and Experimental Therapeutics*, 264 (3): 1198-1205. http://jpet.aspetjournals.org/content/264/3/1198.

Gordon, T. (1993). Factors associated with serum alkaline phosphatase level. *Archives of Pathology & Laboratory Medicine*, 117 (2): 187-190. https://www.ncbi.nlm.nih.gov/pubmed/8427569.

Grassi, G., Seravalle, G., Calhoun, D. A., Bolla, G. B., Giannattasio, C., Marabini, M., and Mancia, G. (1994). Mechanisms responsible for sympathetic activation by cigarette smoking in humans. *Circulation*, 90(1), 248-253. doi: 10.1161/01.cir.90.1.248.

Hart, C. L., Smith, G. D., Gruer, L., and Watt, G. C. (2010). The combined effect of smoking tobacco and drinking alcohol on cause-specific mortality: a 30 year cohort study. *BMC Public Health*, 10 (1): 789. doi: 10.1186/1471-2458-10-789.

Hendriks, H. F. (2007). Moderate alcohol consumption and insulin sensitivity: observations and possible mechanisms. *Annals of Epidemiology*, 17 (5): S40-S42.

Houston, T. K., Person, S. D., Pletcher, M. J., Liu, K., Iribarren, C., and Kiefe, C. I. (2006). Active and passive smoking and development of glucose intolerance among young adults in a prospective cohort: CARDIA study. *BMJ*, 332 (7549): 1064-1069. doi: 10.1136/bmj.38779.584028.55.

Huot, I., Paradis, G., and Ledoux, M. (2004). Factors associated with overweight and obesity in Quebec adults. *International Journal of Obesity*, 28 (6): 766-774. doi: 10.1038/sj.ijo.0802633.

Ilich, J. Z., and Kerstetter, J. E. (2000). Nutrition in bone health revisited: a story beyond calcium. *Journal of the American College of Nutrition*, 19 (6): 715-737. doi: 10.1080/07315724.2000.10718070.

Jatoi, N. A., Jerrard-Dunne, P., Feely, J., and Mahmud, A. (2007). Impact of smoking and smoking cessation on arterial stiffness and aortic wave reflection in hypertension. *Hypertension*, 49 (5): 981-985. doi: 10.1161/HYPERTENSIONAHA.107.087338.

Jessen, A., Buemann, B., Toubro, S., Skovgaard, I. M., and Astrup, A. (2005). The appetite-suppressant effect of nicotine is enhanced by caffeine. *Diabetes, Obesity and Metabolism*, 7 (4): 327-333. doi: 10.1111/j.1463-1326.2004.00389.x.

Jha, P., Jacob, B., Gajalakshmi, V., Gupta, P. C., Dhingra, N., Kumar, R., and Boreham, J. (2008). A nationally representative case–control study of smoking and death in India. *New England Journal of Medicine*, 358 (11): 1137-1147. doi: 10.1056/NEJMsa0707719.

John, U., Hanke, M., Rumpf, H. J., and Thyrian, J. R. (2005). Smoking status, cigarettes per day, and their relationship to overweight and obesity among former and current smokers in a national adult general population sample. *International Journal of Obesity*, 29 (10): 1289-1294. doi: 10.1038/sj.ijo.0803028.

Johnson, R. D., Horowitz, M., Maddox, A. F., Wishart, J. M., and Shearman, D. J. (1991). Cigarette smoking and rate of gastric emptying: effect on alcohol absorption. *BMJ*, 302 (6767): 20-23. doi: 10.1136/bmj.302.6767.20.

Jugdaohsingh, R., O'connell, M. A., Sripanyakorn, S., and Powell, J. J. (2006). Moderate alcohol consumption and increased bone mineral density: potential ethanol and non-ethanol mechanisms. *Proceedings of the Nutrition Society*, 65 (3): 291-310. doi: 10.1079/pns2006508.

Kaczynski, A. T., Manske, S. R., Mannell, R. C., and Grewal, K. (2008). Smoking and physical activity: a systematic review. *American Journal of Health Behavior*, 32 (1): 93-110. doi: 10.5555/ajhb.2008.32.1.93.

Kahn, S. E., Hull, R. L., and Utzschneider, K. M. (2006). Mechanisms linking obesity to insulin resistance and type 2 diabetes. *Nature*, 444 (7121): 840-846. doi: 10.1038/nature05482.

Kapoor, D., and Jones, T. H. (2005). Smoking and hormones in health and endocrine disorders. *European Journal of Endocrinology*, 152 (4): 491-499. doi: https://doi.org/10.1530/eje.1.01867.

Kim, M. J., Shim, M. S., Kim, M. K., Lee, Y., Shin, Y. G., Chung, C. H., and Kwon, S. O. (2003). Effect of chronic alcohol ingestion on bone mineral density in males without liver cirrhosis. *The Korean Journal of Internal Medicine*, 18 (3): 174-180. doi: 10.3904/kjim.2003.18.3.174.

Kim, S. D., Beck, J., Bieniarz, T., Schumacher, A., and Piano, M. R. (2001). A rodent model of alcoholic heart muscle disease and its evaluation by echocardiography. *Alcoholism: Clinical and Experimental Research*, 25 (3): 457-463. doi: https://doi.org/10.1111/j.1530-0277.2001.tb02235.x.

Kiowski, W., Linder, L., Stoschitzky, K., Pfisterer, M., Burckhardt, D., Burkart, F., and Bühler, F. R. (1994). Diminished vascular response to inhibition of endothelium-derived nitric oxide and enhanced vasoconstriction to exogenously administered endothelin-1 in clinically healthy smokers. *Circulation*, 90 (1): 27-34. doi: 10.1161/01.cir.90.1.27.

Kissebah, A. H., and Krakower, G. R. (1994). Regional adiposity and morbidity. *Physiological Reviews*, 74 (4): 761-811. doi: 10.1152/physrev.1994.74.4.761.

Komiyama, M., Wada, H., Ura, S., Yamakage, H., Satoh-Asahara, N., Shimatsu, A. and Hasegawa, K. (2013). Analysis of factors that determine weight gain during smoking cessation therapy. *PloS one*, 8 (8): e72010. doi: 10.1371/journal.pone.0072010.

Koppes, L. L., Dekker, J. M., Hendriks, H. F., Bouter, L. M., and Heine, R. J. (2005). Moderate alcohol consumption lowers the risk of type 2 diabetes. *Diabetes Care*, 28 (3): 719-725. doi: 10.2337/diacare.28.3.719.

Kuriyan, R., Petracchi, C., Ferro-Luzzi, A., Shetty, P. S., and Kurpad, A. V. (1998). Validation of expedient methods for measuring body composition in Indian adults. *The Indian Journal of Medical Research*, 107: 37-45. https://europepmc.org/article/med/9529779.

Landin-Wilhelmsen, K., Wilhelmsen, L., Lappas, G., Rosen, T., Lindstedt, G., Lundberg, P. A. and Bengtsson, B. Å. (1995). Serum intact parathyroid hormone in a random population sample of men and women: relationship to anthropometry, life-style factors, blood pressure, and vitamin D. *Calcified Tissue International*, 56 (2): 104-108. doi: 10.1007/bf00296339.

Lĕ, A. D., Corrigall, W. A., Watchus, J., Harding, S., Juzytsch, W., and Li, T. K. (2000). Involvement of Nicotinic Receptors in Alcohol Self-Administration. *Alcoholism: Clinical and Experimental Research*, 24 (2): 155-163. doi: https://doi.org/10.1111/j.1530-0277.2000.tb04585.x.

Leite, M. L. C., and Nicolosi, A. (2006). Lifestyle correlates of anthropometric estimates of body adiposity in an Italian middle-aged and elderly population: a covariance analysis. *International Journal of Obesity*, 30 (6): 926-934. doi: 10.1038/sj.ijo.0803239.

Lim, S. S., Vos, T., Flaxman, A. D., Danaei, G., Shibuya, K., Adair-Rohani, H. and and Aryee, M. (2012). A comparative risk assessment of burden of disease and injury attributable to 67 risk factors and risk factor clusters in 21 regions, 1990–2010: a systematic analysis for the Global Burden of Disease Study 2010. *The Lancet*, 380 (9859), 2224-2260. doi: 10.1016/S0140-6736(12)61766-8.

Lobo, I. A., and Harris, R. A. (2008). GABA(A) receptors and alcohol. *Pharmacology Biochemistry and Behavior*, 90 (1): 90-94. doi: 10.1016/j.pbb.2008.03.006.

Lourenco, S., Oliveira, A., and Lopes, C. (2012). The effect of current and lifetime alcohol consumption on overall and central obesity. *European Journal of Clinical Nutrition*, 66 (7): 813-818. doi: 10.1038/ejcn.2012.20.

Lukasiewicz, E., Mennen, L. I., Bertrais, S., Arnault, N., Preziosi, P., Galan, P., and Hercberg, S. (2005). Alcohol intake in relation to body mass index and waist-to-hip ratio: the importance of type of alcoholic beverage. *Public Health Nutrition*, 8 (3): 315-320. doi: 10.1079/phn2004680.

Manimunda, S. P., Sugunan, A. P., Thennarasu, K., Pandian, D., Pesala, K. S., and Benegal, V. (2017). Alcohol consumption, hazardous drinking, and alcohol dependency among the population of Andaman and Nicobar Islands, India. *Indian Journal of Public Health*, 61 (2): 105-111. doi: 10.4103/ijph.IJPH_230_15.

Martin, A. D., Spenst, L. F., Drinkwater, D. T., and Clarys, J. P. (1990). Anthropometric estimation of muscle mass in men. *Medicine and Science in Sports and Exercise*, 22 (5): 729-733. doi: 10.1249/00005768-199010000-00027.

Narkiewicz, K., Kjeldsen, S. E., and Hedner, T. (2005). Is smoking a causative factor of hypertension?. *Blood Pressure*, 14 (2): 69-71. doi: 10.1080/08037050510034202.

Pan, A., Wang, Y., Talaei, M., Hu, F. B. and Wu, T. (2015). Relation of active, passive, and quitting smoking with incident type 2 diabetes: a systematic review and meta-analysis. *The Lancet Diabetes & Endocrinology*, 3 (12): 958-967. doi: 10.1016/S2213-8587(15)00316-2.

Panwar, R. B., Gupta, R., Gupta, B. K., Raja, S., Vaishnav, J., Khatri, M., and Agrawal, A. (2011). Atherothrombotic risk factors & premature coronary heart disease in India: a case-control study. *The Indian Journal of Medical Research*, 134 (1): 26-32. http://www.ijmr.org.in/article.asp?issn=0971-5916;year=2011;volume=134;issue=1;spage=26;epage=32;aulast=Panwar.

Pati, S., Swain, S., Mahapatra, S., Hussain, M. A., and Pati, S. (2017). Prevalence, pattern, and correlates of alcohol misuse among male patients attending rural primary care in India. *Journal of Pharmacy & Bioallied Sciences*, 9 (1): 66-72. doi: 10.4103/jpbs.JPBS_325_16.

Peeters, A., Barendregt, J. J., Willekens, F., Mackenbach, J. P., Al Mamun, A., and Bonneux, L. (2003). Obesity in adulthood and its consequences for life expectancy: a life-table analysis. *Annals of Internal Medicine*, 138 (1): 24-32. doi: 10.7326/0003-4819-138-1-200301070-00008.

Perkins, K. A., Epstein, L. H., and Pastor, S. (1990). Changes in energy balance following smoking cessation and resumption of smoking in women. *Journal of Consulting and Clinical Psychology*, 58 (1): 121-125. doi: 10.1037//0022-006x.58.1.121.

Perloff, D., Grim, C., Flack, J., Frohlich, E. D., Hill, M., McDonald, M., and Morgenstern, B. Z. (1993). Human blood pressure determination by sphygmomanometry. *Circulation*, 88 (5): 2460-2470. doi: 10.1161/01.cir.88.5.2460.

Potter, J. F., Watson, R. D., Skan, W., and Beevers, D. G. (1986). The pressor and metabolic effects of alcohol in normotensive subjects. *Hypertension*, 8 (7): 625-631. doi: https://doi.org/10.1161/01.HYP.8.7.625.

Primatesta, P., Falaschetti, E., Gupta, S., Marmot, M. G., and Poulter, N. R. (2001). Association between smoking and blood pressure: evidence from the health survey for England. *Hypertension*, 37 (2): 187-193. doi: 10.1161/01.hyp.37.2.187.

Rajeev, A., Abraham, S. B., Reddy, T. G., Skariah, C. M., Indiradevi, E. R., and Abraham, J. (2017). A community study of alcohol consumption in a rural area of South India. *International Journal of Community Medicine and Public Health*, 4 (6): 2172-2177. doi: http://dx.doi.org/10.18203/2394-6040.ijcmph20172197.

Rehm, J., Baliunas, D., Borges, G. L., Graham, K., Irving, H., Kehoe, T., and Roerecke, M. (2010). The relation between different dimensions of alcohol consumption and burden of disease: an overview. *Addiction*, 105 (5): 817-843. doi: 10.1111/j.1360-0443.2010.02899.x.

Rennie, M. J., Wackerhage, H., Spangenburg, E. E., and Booth, F. W. (2004). Control of the size of the human muscle mass. *Annual Review of Physiology*, 66: 799-828. doi: 10.1146/annurev.physiol.66.052102.134444.

Rimm, E. B., Williams, P., Fosher, K., Criqui, M., and Stampfer, M. J. (1999). Moderate alcohol intake and lower risk of coronary heart disease: meta-analysis of effects on lipids and haemostatic factors. *BMJ*, 319 (7224): 1523-1528. doi: 10.1136/bmj.319.7224.1523.

Rodin, J. (1987). Weight change following smoking cessation: the role of food intake and exercise. *Addictive Behaviors*, 12 (4): 303-317. doi: 10.1016/0306-4603(87)90045-1.

Röjdmark, S., Calissendorff, J., and Brismar, K. (2001). Alcohol ingestion decreases both diurnal and nocturnal secretion of leptin in healthy individuals. *Clinical Endocrinology*, 55 (5): 639-647. doi: 10.1046/ j.1365-2265.2001.01401.x.

Russ, R., Abdel-Rahman, A. R., and Wooles, W. R. (1991). Role of the sympathetic nervous system in ethanol-induced hypertension in rats. *Alcohol*, 8 (4): 301-307. doi: 10.1016/0741-8329(91)90433-w.

Ryu, M., Kimm, H., Jo, J., Lee, S. J., and Jee, S. H. (2010). Association between Alcohol Intake and Abdominal Obesity among the Korean Population. *Epidemiology and Health*, 32, e2010007. doi: 10.4178/epih/e2010007.

Saarni, S. E., Pietiläinen, K., Kantonen, S., Rissanen, A., and Kaprio, J. (2009). Association of smoking in adolescence with abdominal obesity in adulthood: a follow-up study of 5 birth cohorts of Finnish twins. *American Journal of Public Health*, 99 (2): 348-354. doi: 10.2105/ AJPH.2007.123851.

Schrieks, I. C., Heil, A. L., Hendriks, H. F., Mukamal, K. J., and Beulens, J. W. (2015). The effect of alcohol consumption on insulin sensitivity and glycemic status: a systematic review and meta-analysis of intervention studies. *Diabetes Care*, 38 (4): 723-732. doi: 10.2337/dc14-1556.

Sen, A., Das, M., Basu, S., Datta, G. (2015). Prevalence of hypertension and its associated risk factors among Kolkata-based policemen: a sociophysiological study. *International Journal of Medicinal Science and Public Health*. 4 (2): 1-8. doi: 10.5455/ijmsph.2015.0610201444.

Sen, A., Das, M., Basu, S., Datta, G. (2016). Socio-demographic and lifestyle determinants of smokeless tobacco consumption and its association with obesity and hypertension. *Indian Journal of Physiology and Allied Sciences*, 70 (4): 163-176.

Shafey, O., Eriksen, M., Ross, H., & Mackay, J. (2009). *The Tobacco Atlas* 3rd Ed. Atlanta, GA: American Cancer Society; Bookhouse Group.

Shaikh, Z., & Pathak, R. (2017). Revised Kuppuswamy and BG Prasad socio-economic scales for 2016. *International Journal of Community Medicine and Public Health*, 4(4), 997-999.

Siri, W. E. (1956). The gross composition of the body. *Advances in Biological and Medical Physics*, 4 (239-279): 513. doi: 10.1016/b978-1-4832-3110-5.50011-x.

Slagter, S. N., Van Vliet-Ostaptchouk, J. V., Vonk, J. M., Boezen, H. M., Dullaart, R. P., Kobold, A. C. M. and Wolffenbuttel, B. H. (2014). Combined Effects of Smoking and Alcohol on Metabolic Syndrome: The Life Lines Cohort Study. *Plos One*, 9 (4): E96406. doi: 10.1371/journal.pone.0096406.

Slagter, S. N., van Vliet-Ostaptchouk, J. V., Vonk, J. M., Boezen, H. M., Dullaart, R. P., Kobold, A. C. M. and Wolffenbuttel, B. H. (2013). Associations between smoking, components of metabolic syndrome and lipoprotein particle size. *BMC Medicine*, 11 (1): 195. doi: 10.1186/1741-7015-11-195.

Stadler, M., Tomann, L., Storka, A., Wolzt, M., Peric, S., Bieglmayer, C. and Prager, R. (2014). Effects of smoking cessation on β-cell function, insulin sensitivity, body weight, and appetite. *European Journal of Endocrinology*, 170 (2): 219-227. doi: 10.1530/EJE-13-0590.

Sumeet, G., Agrawal, B. K., Sehajpal, P. K., and Goel, R. K. (2011). Prevalence and predictors of essential hypertension in the rural population of Haryana, India: a hospital based study. *Journal of Rural and Tropical Public Health*, 10, 29-34. http://jrtph.jcu.edu.au/vol/JRTPH_Vol10_p29-34_Goel.pdf.

Suter, P. M., and Tremblay, A. (2005). Is alcohol consumption a risk factor for weight gain and obesity? *Critical Reviews in Clinical Laboratory Sciences*, 42 (3): 197-227. doi: https://doi.org/10.1080/10408360590913542.

Talukder, M. H., Johnson, W. M., Varadharaj, S., Lian, J., Kearns, P. N., El-Mahdy, M. A. and Zweier, J. L. (2010). Chronic cigarette smoking causes hypertension, increased oxidative stress, impaired NO bioavailability, endothelial dysfunction, and cardiac remodeling in mice. *American Journal of Physiology-Heart and Circulatory Physiology*, 300 (1): H388-H396. doi: 10.1152/ajpheart.00868.2010.

Tamamizu-Kato, S., Wong, J. Y., Jairam, V., Uchida, K., Raussens, V., Kato, H. and Narayanaswami, V. (2007). Modification by acrolein, a component of tobacco smoke and age-related oxidative stress, mediates functional impairment of human apolipoprotein E. *Biochemistry*, 46 (28): 8392-8400. doi: 10.1021/bi700289k.

Taylor, B., Irving, H. M., Baliunas, D., Roerecke, M., Patra, J., Mohapatra, S., and Rehm, J. (2009). Alcohol and hypertension: gender differences in dose–response relationships determined through systematic review and meta-analysis. *Addiction*, 104 (12): 1981-1990. doi: 10.1111/j.1360-0443.2009.02694.x.

Thompson, W. D., Kelsey, J. L., and Walter, S. D. (1982). Cost and efficiency in the choice of matched and unmatched case-control study designs. *American Journal of Epidemiology*, 116 (5): 840-851. doi: 10.1093/oxfordjournals.aje.a113475.

Thomson, M., Fulton, M., Elton, R. A., Brown, S., Wood, D. A., and Oliver, M. F. (1988). Alcohol consumption and nutrient intake in middle-aged Scottish men. *The American journal of Clinical Nutrition*, 47 (1): 139-145. https://doi.org/10.1093/ajcn/47.1.139.

Trinko, R., Sears, R. M., Guarnieri, D. J., and DiLeone, R. J. (2007). Neural mechanisms underlying obesity and drug addiction. *Physiology & Behavior*, 91 (5): 499-505. doi: 10.1016/j.physbeh.2007.01.001.

van de Wiel, A. (2004). Diabetes mellitus and alcohol. *Diabetes/ Metabolism Research and Reviews*, 20 (4): 263-267. doi: https://doi.org/10.1002/dmrr.492.

Vary, T. C., and Lang, C. H. (2008). Assessing effects of alcohol consumption on protein synthesis in striated muscles. In *Alcohol* (pp. 343-355). Humana Press.

Vasdev, S., Sampson, C. A., and Prabhakaran, V. M. (1991). Platelet-free calcium and vascular calcium uptake in ethanol-induced hypertensive rats. *Hypertension*, 18 (1): 116-122. doi: https://doi.org/10.1161/01.HYP.18.1.116.

Venkataraman, R., Satish Kumar, B. P., Kumaraswamy, M., Singh, R., Pandey, M., and Tripathi, P. (2013). Smoking, alcohol and hypertension. *International Journal of Pharmacy and Pharmaceutical Sciences*, 5 (4): 28-32.

Vestergaard, P., and Mosekilde, L. (2003). Fracture risk associated with smoking: a meta-analysis. *Journal of Internal Medicine*, 254 (6): 572-583. doi: https://doi.org/10.1111/j.1365-2796.2003.01232.x.

Wang, G. J., Volkow, N. D., Logan, J., Pappas, N. R., Wong, C. T., Zhu, W. and Fowler, J. S. (2001). Brain dopamine and obesity. *The Lancet*, 357 (9253): 354-357. doi: 10.1016/s0140-6736(00)03643-6.

Weiderpass, E. (2010). Lifestyle and cancer risk. *Journal of Preventive Medicine and Public Health*, 43 (6): 459-471. doi: 10.3961/jpmph.2010.43.6.459.

World Health Organization. (2000). International association for the study of obesity, international obesity task force. *The Asia-Pacific perspective: redefining obesity and its treatment*, 15-21. https://apps.who.int/iris/handle/10665/206936.

World Health Organization. (2009). *WHO Report on the Global Tobacco Epidemic*, 2009: Implementing Smoke-free Environments. Geneva: World Health Organization. https://www.who.int/tobacco/mpower/2009/gtcr_download/en/.

World Health Organization. (2013). WHO STEPwise approach to chronic disease risk factor surveillance-Instrument v2.0. Department of Chronic Diseases and Health Promotion. *World Health Organization*, 20. https://www.who.int/ncds/surveillance/steps/Grenada_2010-11_STEPS_Report.pdf.

World Health Organization. (2016). *Global status report on alcohol and health* 2014. Geneva: WHO; 2014. https://apps.who.int/iris/bitstream/handle/10665/112736/9789240692763_eng.pdf;jsessionid=DFB76E1F55105A4F5F5882B7AF4DB965?sequence=1.

Yanbaeva, D. G., Dentener, M. A., Creutzberg, E. C., Wesseling, G., & Wouters, E. F. (2007). Systemic effects of smoking. *Chest*, 131 (5): 1557-1566. doi: 10.1378/chest.06-2179.

Yeomans, M. R. (2010). Short term effects of alcohol on appetite in humans. Effects of context and restrained eating. *Appetite*, 55 (3): 565-573. doi: 10.1016/j.appet.2010.09.005.

Yeomans, M. R., & Gray, R. W. (2002). Opioid peptides and the control of human ingestive behaviour. *Neuroscience & Biobehavioral Reviews*, 26 (6): 713-728. doi: 10.1016/s0149-7634(02)00041-6.

Zhang, S., Liu, Y., Wang, G., Xiao, X., Gang, X., Li, F. and Wang, G. (2016). The relationship between alcohol consumption and incidence of glycometabolic abnormality in middle-aged and elderly Chinese men. *International Journal of Endocrinology*, 2016. doi: https://doi.org/10.1155/2016/1983702.

In: West Bengal
Editor: Rhianu Bowell

ISBN: 978-1-53619-237-7
© 2021 Nova Science Publishers, Inc.

*Chapter 2*

# MGNREGA AND WOMEN EMPOWERMENT: SOCIO-ECONOMIC IMPLICATIONS

## *Arindam Chakraborty*[*]
Sudhiranjan Lahiri Mahavidyalaya, West Bengal, India

### ABSTRACT

The Mahatma Gandhi National Rural Employment Guarantee Act (MGNREGA) was initiated in India in 2006 with a view to creating more wage employment in rural areas thereby ameliorating rural poverty. With the right based framework and demand-driven approach, its initial target has been to guarantee at least 100 days of employment to adults of the rural households every year. But after the completion of more than a decade, the effects and roles of the scheme are found to be manifolds. Particularly, if we consider the impact of women participation under the scheme the results can be witnessed in varied fields. As the scheme has converted some of the unpaid hours of the women into paid hours it has started to change their role in the family. By putting cash in the hands of women MGNREGA has allowed them greater bargaining power in the family thereby diversifying the contributions that women have been making to households. There have been drastic changes in the family

---

[*] Corresponding Author's E-mail: arindamfulia@gmail.com.

consumption pattern as well as family budgeting. While their contribution to the health account has augmented economic security, their role as a financier of the children for their education has led to substantial changes, even impacting the school dropout rate to some extent. All these issues have been taken care of in this chapter based on a micro-level survey done in the district of Nadia, West Bengal.

**Keywords**: MGNREGA, bargaining power, family spending, education, wastage problem

## INTRODUCTION

The policy initiative of the Government of India in terms of Mahatma Gandhi National Rural Employment Guarantee Act (hereinafter MGNREGA1) has been conceived primarily to alleviate poverty by providing households with a guaranteed income through employment on public projects. The scheme seeks to provide basic social security to India's rural poor and provides 100 days of guaranteed wage employment to every rural household. Although it is not a women empowerment programme, it is inherently sensitive to the issues of gender discrimination in the labour market. It aims at increasing and improving rural women's labour market opportunities (Afridi, Mukhopadhyaya & Sahoo 2012). There are several provisions in the Act such as 33 percent reservation for the women workers, equal wages for both men and women, childcare facilities (crèche facility) at the worksites which are of special interest to women workers. The gender-friendly design of the scheme has certainly facilitated women's participation and enhanced their share of the benefits (Carswell & De Neve 2013). It can help empower women by giving them independent income-earning opportunities (Dreze 2011).

In the discussion of development policy, it is often argued that income generation of women as a means of reduction of poverty ensures them

---

[1] Initially, it was the National Rural Employment Guarantee Act (NREGA). From October 2, 2009, NREGA has been rechristened as Mahatma Gandhi National Rural Employment Guarantee Act (re-acronym as MGNREGA).

greater bargaining power within the household which in turn impacts intra-household decision making, family spending on food, health, education and other (Afridi et al. 2012). As the women are getting handsomely benefitted out of the scheme with the enhanced share it is expected to unleash a change in the pattern of family spending as reflected in the previous study that significant increase in women's paid work has led to improvement in food consumption in certain sections of society (Chandrasekhar & Ghosh 2009). The chapter basically emphasizes the impact of the scheme on family spending in general and on school dropout in particular, in the perspective of greater bargaining power of the women attained due to the scheme.

## DATA AND METHODOLOGY

The findings of this chapter are based on an extensive survey carried out at the household level in the 2016-17 financial year in eight gram panchayats (village panchayats) selected randomly from four blocks of Nadia district of West Bengal. In the study, a multi-stage sampling procedure was followed. In the very first stage, district Nadia was selected purposively as it topped the list among 19 MGNREGA districts of the State in the performance ranking made by the State MGNREGA cell on the basis of 11 parameters[2] in 2015-16. It was expected that the top-ranking district would deliver excellence in most of the fields. In Nadia, there were 17 blocks in 2015-16. In the second stage, out of them, four blocks such as Chakdaha, Krishnaganj, Nakasipara and Santipur were selected randomly. From these four blocks, eight gram panchayat were chosen randomly again in the third stage taking two panchayats from each block. Now from our data, it reveals that Hingnara and Sarati from Chakdaha, Bhajanghat-Tungi

---

[2] Parameters are: Percentage of person-days generated against last year performance; Average person-days per household; % of household completed 100 days; % of work with convergence; Work completion rate; % of SC/ST households provided employment against registered SC/ST; % of wage paid within 15 days; Women % of person-days; Expenditure (in Lakh); % of less than15 days employment provided against household provided employment; % of Aadhaar Number w.r.t active workers.

and Taldah Majdia from Krishnaganj, Birpur-II and Patikabari from Nakasipara and Belgoria-I and Fulia Township from Santipur blocks were selected for our purpose. In the fourth stage, villages were selected randomly taking one or two villages from each of the panchayats. In the last stage, 500 odd households working in the MGNREGA works were selected from these villages, but the target was to reach to the female workers only.

## SOCIO-ECONOMIC PROFILE

This section of the chapter deals with the presentation and analysis of micro-level data. In Table 1 profile of the sample has been presented. Regarding caste it has revealed that there were 15.2 percent of general category women, 36.2 percent belonged to Scheduled Castes (SC) consisting of more than $1/3^{rd}$ of the sample, 28 percent belonged to Scheduled Tribes (ST) and the remaining 20.6 percent were from OBCa (Other Backward Classes) category. Regarding the religion of the sample women, it was observed that the data were lopsided to the Hindu community with almost $4/5^{th}$ of the women hailing from this community. Samples having Muslim women were centred only to two panchayats namely; Sarati panchayat of Chakdaha block and Birpur-II panchayat of Nakasipara block while the remaining six samples contained Hindu community women.

In general, the women in the sample had a lower literacy rate. Only 41.4 percent of women were literate. Among literate women, Fulia Township panchayat of Santipur block housed the highest number of them with almost $3/4^{th}$ of its women workers in the sample numbering 72 being literate. There was more illiteracy among the ST women with 87.1 percent being illiterate among them.

## Table 1. Profile of the women workers

| Category | % |
|---|---|
| Gen | 15.2 |
| SC | 36.2 |
| ST | 28 |
| OBC$_a$ | 20.6 |
| Hindu | 79.4 |
| Muslim | 20.6 |
| Illiterate | 58.6 |
| APL | 41.4 |
| BPL | 58.6 |
| IAY | 14.6 |

Source: Primary data.

On the economic front, apart from some other issues, the study has tried to amass data on the poverty level of the selected households. Poverty can be defined as the inability of an individual to secure a normative minimum level of living or to attain some basic needs of life. This normative minimum defines the poverty line in terms of money per capita per month living below which a person is deemed to be poor (Planning Commission 2014). On the poverty account, the study has collected data on three heads, namely APL, BPL, and the IAY[3] beneficiary. Around 58.6 percent of women in the sample hailed from BPL families out of which 73 families consisting of 14.6 percent of the total households received the IAY benefit as they were poor to a considerable extent. This reflects that in most cases we have been able to reach the women for whom the scheme has been designed.

In the study, in presenting the workers by their age, the age group has been divided into four classes in Table 2. All the women in the sample were scattered in the different age groups. Almost half of the workers were from the age group 31-45 years comprising of 46 percent. In the sample, 7.4 percent of workers were above 60 years of age. This is a picture showing the willingness of the workers of different ages to be engaged in

---

[3] Indira Awas Yojana (IAY), a flagship scheme of the Ministry of Rural Development, Govt. of India provides assistance to BPL families who are either houseless or having inadequate housing facilities for constructing a safe and durable shelter.

the work. What is most interesting is that even women over 60 years of age also vied for MGNREGA works as revealed by the data. This indicates two aspects. On one hand, women having age more than 60 years had to struggle for their survival due to their abject penury. In some of the worksites, they did the job of water carriers, but most of the senior women had to work hard even carrying the soil for earning the wage, if not digging. The other case tells that the scheme has created a space even for the senior women to work for their livelihood which is hardly found in other schemes. This is no doubt the uniqueness of the scheme.

**Table 2. Women workers by age**

| Age-Groups | % |
|---|---|
| 18-30 yrs | 18.8 |
| 31-45 yrs | 46 |
| 46-60 yrs | 27.8 |
| 60+ yrs | 7.4 |
| Total | 100 |

Source: Primary data.

## MGNREGA PARTICIPATION

As the chapter deals with the socio-economic implications of MGNREGA in respect of the participation of women, it is pertinent to present the scenario of their participation under the scheme. In this chapter, to get a wider scenario regarding women participation under the scheme, the average participation of the sample women under MGNREGA for the last three years has been considered instead of only one year as done by earlier studies (Khera & Nayek 2009; Pankaj & Tankha 2010). As the survey was done in 2016-17, the average number of days of employment enjoyed by the women under the scheme during the last three financial year i.e 2013-14, 2014-15, 2015-16 has been considered here. Considering the aggregate data, it can be stated that around 69 percent of women in the sample enjoyed on average 31-100 days of job under the scheme during the last three years, the majority being in the working bracket 31-60 days with around 48.2 percent women having received work to that extent. It implies that the remaining 31 percent, almost 1/3$^{rd}$ of the women in the sample, received only 0- 30 days of employment under the scheme during the period. However, the number of women enjoyed 100 days of employment throughout the period pegged at only three. They were the workers in Sarati panchayat of Chakdaha block entrusted with ICDS job in terms of cleaning and sweeping of the local school campus for the last three years.

## IMPACT ON FAMILY SPENDING

When women are put into productive activities their paid hours result in a change in the consumption pattern of the family by directly affecting the family expenditure. Our employment data show that around 69 percent of women in the sample worked between 31-100 days on average during the last three financial years under the scheme. It implies that MGNREGA ensured handsome income to village womenfolk during the last three years as far as our study is concerned. It is then obvious that this earning would have some immediate effects on the family spending of the women under the sample. These impacts have been coined as 'Social and Economic Benefits' of MGNREGA by Khera & Nayek (2009). Jandu (2008) has also dealt with this dimension in his study. Our survey in this behalf reflects some interesting findings.

In the time of the survey, the questions on family spending considered seven avenues through which women spent their wage-income namely avoiding hunger, avoiding illness, schooling of children, fulfilling personal needs, creating assets, repaying debts and savings. The responses are drafted in Table 3. Interestingly most of the women opted for two avenues, one was avoiding hunger and the other was the schooling of their children. In aggregate 50.6 percent of women replied that MGNREGA employment enabled them to face less hunger. In Taldah Majdia panchayat of Krishnagnaj block where 93.8 percent of families in the sample were living below the poverty line, 78.1 percent of women opted for this avenue, the highest percentage among the lot. It transpires from Table 1 that in aggregate around 58.6 percent of families were living below the so-called poverty level. Apart from this, 241 numbers of women consisting of 48.2 percent of the sample opined that poverty was the prime driving force for opting MGNREGA. So, on this ground, this response is very much expected.

Another interesting response is the spending of MGNREGA money on the schooling of children. Our survey data show that 48 percent of women in the sample spent money on this account. Now from our data, it transpires that in aggregate around 60 percent of the family had school-going children. The scheme helped them a lot to purchase the books or other items required and to pay the tuition fees of the private tutors of their children.

The scheme has also acted as the 'healthline' (Khera & Nayek 2009) for many rural households. Around 30 percent of women reported using the MGNREGA wage for treatment of illness of the family members or of their own either in the form of sudden or chronic ailments. In Hingnara panchayat of Chakdaha block, some of the women reported that their family members had been suffering from water-borne diseases as the water quality there was very poor. So suffering from bowel problems such as gas, acidity, indigestion was a common phenomenon in almost all families. There 30.6 percent of women replied that a bulk of MGNREGA wage was spent on medical account. Similarly, in Birpur-II panchayat of Nakasipara block, several ailments were found in the sample women hailing from the Muslim community because of their unhygienic living in shabby dwellings, with 65 percent of workers in the sample living in Hut or Tiled rooms. In this panchayat, 38.3 percent of women spent their MGNREGA earnings for treatment of their family members including themselves.

In Sarati panchayat of Chakdaha, Bhajanghat-Tungi panchayat of Krishnaganj and Belgoria-I panchayat of Santipur blocks, it was observed that respectively 39.5, 37.4 and 33.3 percent of women spent their wages on health account. It has been reflected in the survey that in these three panchayats from 42.5 to 51.5 percent women workers were aged about 46 years and above while in some other panchayats having fewer aged women workers it was found to be comparably less expenditure on medical purpose. It implies that a sample having a higher number of aged women spent more on the medical ground out of their MGNREGA earnings. So, it can be stated that in most cases older women opted for the avenue of medical expenses for spending their MGNREGA wages as they or their husbands used to suffer from many age-related diseases.

**Table 3. Effects on family spending**

| Blocks | Gram Panchayats | Proportion (%) of women workers who spent MGNREGA earnings to | | | | | | |
|---|---|---|---|---|---|---|---|---|
| | | Avoid Hunger | Avoid Illness | Schooling of Children | Personal needs | Create Assets | Repay Debts | Savings |
| Chakdaha | Hingnara | 40.3 | 30.6 | 40.3 | 9.7 | 9.7 | 1.4 | 8.3 |
| | Sarati | 76.7 | 39.5 | 53.5 | 18.6 | 00 | 00 | 00 |
| Krishnaganj | Bhajanghat Tungi | 43.4 | 37.4 | 35.5 | 27.3 | 20.2 | 02 | 00 |
| | Taldah Majdia | 78.1 | 21.9 | 21.9 | 3.1 | 00 | 00 | 00 |
| Nakasipara | Birpur-II | 71.7 | 38.3 | 41.7 | 6.7 | 1.7 | 1.7 | 00 |
| | Patikabari | 67.2 | 23.4 | 65.6 | 28.1 | 6.2 | 00 | 1.6 |
| Santipur | Belgoria-I | 42.4 | 33.3 | 48.5 | 48.5 | 03 | 9.1 | 00 |
| | Fulia Township | 23.7 | 18.6 | 64.9 | 23.7 | 10.3 | 17.5 | 9.3 |
| Total | | 50.6 | 30 | 48 | 20.8 | 8.6 | 4.8 | 3.2 |

Source: Primary data.

In some cases, womens pent some of their earnings for their own needs. Around 20.8 percent women replied that they spent their earnings for the purchase of their garments, usual cosmetic items, for going out of home, so on and so forth. When women received handsome income out of employment under the scheme, after meeting some basic needs they also opted for assets creation, repaying debts or savings. Around 8.6 percent of women in the sample were able to create assets out of MGNREGA earnings, the type and quality of which varied across the panchayats in the form of boring tube-well, purchasing a Gas oven, cattle, jewelry or furniture or making kitchen or toilet or rooftop of IAY construction and the likes.

In Fulia Township panchayat of Santipur block, a lot of women were the members of Self-Help Groups. For various reasons, they had to take loans. A significant percentage of workers (around 17.5 percent) of this panchayat replied that they were able to repay the loans with the help of MGNREGA wages. In some other panchayats also women repaid loans out of MGNREGA wages, taken for making room or purchase of land. On savings account, it was seen that some of the women in Hingnara panchayat of Chakdaha block and Fulia Township panchayat of Santipur block were able to save a part of their wages and utilised it for cultivation in their own or lease land. Previously in some cases, this cultivation was done by taking loans from local moneylenders. But they came out to be self-sufficient to some extent in financing the cultivation of their small tracks of land due to the scheme.

## IMPACT ON SCHOOL DROPOUT

Although women spend a lot of time for household maintenance, management and shopping for own family, care for children, the sick, elderly as well as for different minor productive activities, their contribution to the household income and the national economy remains largely unaccounted for (Pankaj & Tankha 2010). This is because their works are generally unpaid. The MGNREGA has opened up an opportunity for going outside of the home for productive purposes for which they are paid for, all the women in general and around 60 percent of women in our sample who did not have any other involvement apart from their household chores. The scheme has converted some of their unpaid hours of work into paid hours of work. Participation of the women under MGNREGA and thereby converting unpaid hours of work into paid hours of work has ushered in greater bargaining power of women within the household which has been reflected in the family budgeting in general in the previous part of this chapter.

Focusing on the education aspect it was seen that in the study nearly 50 percent of women responded to spend their wages for the education of their wards. It has been reflected in the previous study that greater participation of women in MGNREGA works has a positive impact on the children's time in school (Afridi et al. 2012). As far as our survey is concerned we have got nearly 60 percent of families having school-going children and 36 percent families having school-going children more than one in number as reflected from Table 4. The Table also presents the average school-going children per household and the rate of dropout of the sample households. In aggregate there have been 1.04 average school-going children per household in the sample. In the study, the rate of dropout has been assessed by taking the ratio of the total number of children dropped out of the school system with the total number of dropped out plus school-going children and multiplying it by 100. In aggregate we have got a 10.53 percent dropout rate for some 61 children in 41 households which is no doubt a considerable figure for a small sample like ours.

**Table 4. School going and dropout children of the women workers**

| Block | Chakdaha | | Krishnaganj | | Nakasipara | | Santipur | | Total |
|---|---|---|---|---|---|---|---|---|---|
| Gram Panchayats/Numbers | Hingnara | Sarati | Bhajanghat Tungi | Taldah Majdia | Birpur-II | Patikabari | Belgoria-I | Fulia Township | |
| Nil | 32 (44.4) | 17 (39.5) | 45 (45.4) | 24 (75) | 22 (36.7) | 14 (21.9) | 15 (45.5) | 32 (33) | 201 (40.2) |
| 1 | 16 (22.2) | 14 (32.6) | 29 (29.3) | 03 (9.4) | 13 (21.7) | 16 (25) | 08 (24.2) | 20 (20.6) | 119 (23.8) |
| 2 | 22 (30.6) | 10 (23.3) | 19 (19.2) | 03 (9.4) | 18 (30) | 27 (42.2) | 09 (27.3) | 38 (39.2) | 146 (29.2) |
| 3 and more | 2 (2.8) | 02 (4.6) | 06 (6.1) | 02 (6.2) | 07 (11.6) | 07 (10.9) | 01 (03) | 07 (7.2) | 34 (6.8) |
| Total School-going Children | 66 (13.2) | 40 (08) | 82 (16.4) | 16 (3.2) | 72 (15.4) | 95 (19) | 29 (5.8) | 118 (23.6) | 518 (100) |
| Average School-going Children per HH | 0.92 | 0.93 | 0.82 | 0.5 | 1.2 | 1.48 | 0.87 | 1.21 | 1.04 |
| Dropout Households | 01 (2.4) | 08 (19.5) | 06 (14.6) | 09 (21.9) | 10 (24.5) | 02 (4.8) | 01 (2.4) | 04 (9.8) | 41 (100) |
| Total Dropout Children | 01 (1.6) | 12 (19.7) | 11 (18) | 15 (24.6) | 13 (21.3) | 04 (6.6) | 01 (1.6) | 04 (6.6) | 61 (100) |
| Dropout Rate | 1.5 | 23.1 | 11.8 | 48.4 | 15.9 | 4.1 | 3.3 | 3.3 | 10.53 |

Note: In the parentheses, percentages are given. Source: Primary data.

It has been the objective of the study to find out the factors affecting the rate of dropout in the study area. Does higher participation of women under the scheme leave any impact on children's dropout? In order to determine the factors impacting the school dropout, logistic regression has been attempted in the study where the response variable school dropout is considered to be a binary one where dropout =1 if yes, otherwise=0. We assume the following logistic equation:

$$L = \log(p/1-p) = \beta_0 + \beta_1 X_1 + \beta_2 X_2 + \beta_3 X_3 + u_i \qquad (1)$$

where p is the probability of school dropout and

$X_1$= Women Workers Religion where Hindu=1, otherwise=0
$X_2$= Poverty Level, where BPL=1, otherwise=0
$X_3$= Women Workers 3 Years Average Participation in MGNREGA
and $u_i$ is the error term.

Based on the survey data, estimates of the binary logistic regression equation (1) have been computed using STATA 12. The results of the logistic analysis for school dropout are drafted in Table 5. The Table presents the estimated coefficients, marginal effects and odds ratio for various co-variates under study. The results describe the relationship between the independent variables and the response variable, where the response variable is on the logit scale.

**Table 5. Results of logistic regression on school dropout**

| Variables | Coefficients | z | Odds Ratio | Marginal effects | z |
|---|---|---|---|---|---|
| Constant | -0.981(0.528) | -1.86 | 0.903(0.198) | | |
| $X_1$ | -1.172*(0.342) | -3.42 | 0.309* (0.106) | -0.093*(0.034) | -2.72 |
| $X_2$ | 0.728**(0.372) | 1.96 | 2.071**(0.769) | 0.04**(0.019) | 2.03 |
| $X_3$ | -0.027*(0.009) | -2.75 | 0.973*(0.009) | -0.002*(0.001) | -3.14 |

Note: Standard errors are in parentheses.
LR chi2(3) = 25.88 Prob > chi2= 0.0000.
*Significant at 1% & ** Significant at 5% level.
Source: Primary Data.

All the three coefficients of the explanatory variables have come out to be highly significant here. Considering the significant religion coefficient it reveals that the rate of dropout is found to be more prevalent among the Muslims in the study. It increases the likelihood of drop out by 9.3 percentage points. In both of the samples having Muslim women in Sarati panchayat of Chakdaha block and Birpur-II panchayat of Nakasipara block, the dropout cases were found in a higher number of households (19.5 percent in Sarati and 24.5 Percent in Birpur-II) in comparison to other panchayats excepting Taldah Majdia panchayat in Krishnaganj block with 21.6 percent. The lower annual income of the families might be one of the reasons here as it has been revealed from our data that in Birpur-II panchayat annual income of 78.3 percent of families were found to be in the range of Rs 0-30000 (excluding MGNREGA income) in 2015-16, the highest percentage among the panchayats in the study.

The significant positive coefficient for poverty level implies that women living below the poverty level have experienced a higher rate of dropout, for every one-unit increase in poverty, we expect a 2.071 times increase in the odds of school dropout. Poverty disallows people to be well-fed, well-nourished, well educated, so on and so forth. It debars people from having the basic capabilities. It has been found to be true in our study too reflecting more dropout cases among the women workers who were living below the poverty line.

Considering the coefficient of MGNREGA participation of women it can be stated that for every one-unit increase in MGNREGA participation of women, we expect a 0.972 times decrease in the odds of school dropout. Higher female participation under the scheme has had a negative impact on school dropout as far as our data is concerned. So, the employment generation of women under MGNREGA turns out to be a good answer to the dropout problem in the study areas.

## Conclusion

By its design MGNREGA is inherently sensitive to women's participation under the scheme thereby increasing employment opportunities for rural women. As a result of MGNREGA, increased income has ensured a greater degree of economic independence among women (Jandu 2008). Higher employment opportunities under the scheme have led to higher income generation to women ushering in a greater degree of economic independence among women which in turn has impacted intra-household decision making, family spending on food, health, education, and others. Wages earned by women from the scheme have found several avenues to be disposed of which have been reflected in the family budgeting of the beneficiary households.

In the case of more than 50 percent of the sample households, the scheme has enabled them to face less hunger by allowing them to have two square meals. In Bhajanghat-Tungi panchayat, Annabala Bag or Haridasi Sardar, both septuagenarian widows, used to earn a livelihood by other's help or sometimes they collected fruits and vegetables from jungles and fields for their subsistence. In Birpur-II panchayat, Rahima Bibi, aged 60 years, with his feeble husband had no other way to earn a livelihood than to depend on other's help. They were the representatives of so many in the sample used to earn a livelihood in these crude ways. To them, MGNREGA emerged as God's mercy which had enabled them to live in the society with their head held high. So, in one way it has ensured the basic entitlement to the rural people that has enabled them to be well-fed and well-nourished and to mingle in the social life with dignity. In another way, in the context of ensuring food security in rural areas, it has come out to be an effective instrument to some extent.

Wages spent by women on health purposes for the treatment of illness of the family members or their own either in the form of sudden or chronic ailments have unfolded two important dimensions. In most cases, there is a strong relationship between keeping fit and taking part in the economic activities. The MGNREGA income has enabled them to keep fit for work to some extent. So, in respect of the augmenting economic security of the rural womenfolk the scheme has proved to be playing an important role (Khera & Nayek 2009). Secondly, there have been several cases where older women opted for this avenue of medical expenses for spending the bulk of their MGNREGA wage-income as they or their husbands used to suffer from many age-related diseases. In Birpur-II panchayat, Anawara Bibi, aged 61 years spent a bulk of wages for treatment of her ailing husband or Kuruni Bewa, 62 years widow living alone was able to see the doctor only because of MGNREGA earning. In this way, the scheme has offered a new meaning of life to the older womenfolk of the rural areas and truly made their life worth living.

Apart from meeting necessities, wage-earning has also allowed the sample households for opting for creating some assets as a means of necessary or as a luxury, repaying debts or saving a part of income depending on the days of employment they enjoyed as well as the belongings they already had. When they used MGNREGA wages for boring tube-well, purchasing furniture, making kitchen or toilet or supplementing IAY construction for rooftop it might be considered as their necessary asset creation while expenditure on jewelry was surely a luxury they could afford with wages. In Patikabari panchayat, Jasodha Sarkar, a 62 years old woman purchased gold earrings out of wages. Apart from her old age pension, she enjoyed on average 95 days of work under the scheme during the last three years.

The scheme has also initiated the savings habit among women workers. In Patikabari panchayat, Ramala Biswas hailing from a BPL family was paying LIC premium out of wage-earnings. Apart from this, women were able to save a part of their wage-earnings and utilised it for repaying SHG loans or loans taken for making room or purchase of land. Even they used their MGNREGA earnings for cultivation in their own or lease land. Previously money required for this sort of purpose was met by taking a loan from a local moneylender. They no longer needed to go to the moneylenders. Income from the scheme helped them to be emancipated them from the noose of indebtedness. They came out to be self-sufficient in financing the cultivation of their small tracks of land. It helped them keep themselves away from the clutches of local moneylenders (Jandu

2008). MGNREGA by making them less dependent on debt from moneylenders has enabled them to live life with more peace and dignity.

The impact of MGNREGA on education can be envisaged from two dimensions; first, as a source of finance for giving education to children in rural areas and secondly, as a solution to the wastage[4] problem of the education sector as well. Nearly 50 percent of women responded to spend their wages on the education of their children. In the study, families having school-going children used the wages for the continuation of schooling of their children by purchasing books or other items required and paying the tuition fees to the private tutors of their children. So, the scheme has emerged as a good financier for educating the rural children of the study areas.

In the logit analysis dropout cases have significantly found to be more prevalent among women hailing from the Muslim community. The lower annual income of the family has revealed to be one of the reasons for more prevalence of the problem among Muslim women of the study. So, putting more Muslim women in the job of the scheme can spell a good answer to the persistent problem of school dropout among them.

Poverty accounts for the deepening of the dropout problem in rural areas. It disallows the people from having the basic capability of being well educated. Our study has reflected more dropout cases among the children of the women workers who were living below the poverty line. On the contrary, higher women participation under the scheme has revealed to have a lessening impact on school dropout. From the policy point of view this is a very crucial finding. When women are self-sufficient enough to ensure the education of their children, they enjoy greater bargaining power in intra-household decision making. They can voice for sending their children to school instead of keeping them at home doing nothing or putting them into work.This fact ushers in a greater impact on school dropout. This finding vouches for more employment generation among rural women through the scheme. Secondly, as the MGNREGA has been devised to ameliorate rural poverty, the more employment will be

---

[4] Wastage is defined as the premature withdrawal of pupils from school at any stage before completion of the course (Purkait, 2005).

generated the higher the rate at which poverty will be arrested. So, higher MGNREGA employment would not only help ameliorate poverty but ultimately result in curbing the wastage problem in the education sector in rural areas.

All these taken together, it seems that MGNREGA is making a major shift in the role of women in the family by way of conversion of some of their unpaid hours into paid hours. Women are no longer mere spectators in the family, rather taking active roles in every dimension of family matters. In the process of empowerment, one of the important ingredients is the decision making in the family (Garba 1999; Alkire et al. 2013) which has been duly fostered by the MGNREGA work opportunities. By putting the cash in the hands of women MGNREGA has allowed them greater bargaining power in the family thereby diversifying the contributions that women have been making to households (Jandu 2008). By ensuring the increased income in the hands of women MGNREGA has started to create a new hope among the rural womenfolk. It allows them to believe that they will not have to sleep hungry; they can see the doctors if requires; their children's education will not stop in the midway; they will not have to survive with other's help. MGNREGA has reached them to a new horizon where they can heave a sigh of relief. This is the true outcome of the scheme in the socio-economic field.

## REFERENCES

Afridi, F., Mukhopadhyaya, A., & Sahoo, S. (2012). *Female labour force participation and child education in India: The effect of the national rural employment guarantee scheme.* Discussion Paper No. 6593, IZA, Germany. Retrieved from http://ftp.iza.org/dp6593.pdf on 08.08.2016.

Alkire, S., Meinzen-Dick, R., Peterman, A., Quisumbing, A., Seymour, G., & Vaz, A. (2013). The women's empowerment in agriculture index, *World Development,* 52, 71–91. http://dx.doi.org/10.1016/j.worlddev.2013.06.007.

Carswell, G., & De Neve, G. (2013). Women at the crossroads: Implementation of employment guarantee scheme in rural Tamil Nadu. *Economic and Political Weekly*, 68(52), 82-93.

Chandrasekhar, C.P., & Ghosh, J. (2009). Social inclusion in the NREGS. *Business Line*, January, 27, 2009. Retrieved from https://www.the hindubusinessline.com/todays-paper/tp-opinion/Social-inclusion-in-the-NREGS/article20084108.ece on 12.09.11.

Dreze, J. (2011). Employment guarantee and right to work. In R. Khera (Ed.) *The battle for employment guarantee* (pp. 03-20). New Delhi: Oxford University Press.

Garba, P. K. (1999). An endogenous empowerment strategy: a case-study of Nigerian women. *Development in Practice*, 9(I & 2), February 1999, 130-141.

Jandu, N. (2008). Employment guarantee and women empowerment in rural India. Retrieved from *www.righttoffodindia.or*on 30.06.2014.

Khera, R., & Nayak, N. (2009). Women workers and perceptions of the national rural employment guarantee act. *Economic and Political Weekly*, 44(43), 49-57.

Pankaj, A., & Tankha, R. (2010). Empowerment effects of the NREGS on women workers: A study in four states. *Economic and Political Weekly*, 45(30), 45-55.

Planning Commission, Government of India. (2014). *Report of the expert group to review the methodology for measurement of poverty*. Retrieved from http://planningcommission.nic.in/reports/genrep/pov_rep0707.pdf on 02.03.16.

Purkait, B. R. (2005). *Milestones in modern Indian education*, India: New Central Book Agency (P) Ltd.

In: West Bengal
Editor: Rhianu Bowell

ISBN: 978-1-53619-237-7
© 2021 Nova Science Publishers, Inc.

*Chapter 3*

# AGE TRENDS IN ANTHROPOMETRIC CHARACTERISTICS AND NUTRITIONAL STATUS AMONG ADULT MAHALI FEMALES OF BANKURA DISTRICT, WEST BENGAL, INDIA

*Kaushik Bose\*, PhD, DSc, Shilpita Bhandar[1], Mihir Ghosh, PhD, Binoy Kumar Kuiti, PhD Soma Pal and Swarup Pratihar*
[1]Department of Anthropology, Vidyasagar University, Midnapore, West Bengal, India

## ABSTRACT

The present study was undertaken to assess age trends in anthropometric measures and nutritional status among adult Mahali females. It was a community-based cross-sectional study, carried out in

---

\* Corresponding Author's E-mail: kaushikbose@cantab.net.

selected four villages of Bankura district, West Bengal, India. A total of 118 Mahali tribals, aged over 18 years were included in our study. The participants were further classified into three age groups: $\leq 30$ years, 31-49 years, $\geq 50$ years. Anthropometric variables included height, weight, sitting height, knee height, mid-upper arm, medial calf circumferences and body mass index (BMI). In general, an inverse age trend was observed in all these anthropometric variables. This age trend was statistically significant ($p < 0.05$) in case of height, weight, sitting height and medial calf circumference. In nutritional assessment, 75 individuals were found to have chronic energy deficiency (CED). This could have serious health implications.

**Keywords**: Age, Body Mass Index, Nutritional Status

## INTRODUCTION

Changes in body structure and morphology in humans occurs over a lifetime. At every stage of life, there are physical changes in the human body. Although every person experiences growth and development uniquely, the patterns are similar for all humans but the rates vary (due to nutrition, daily work activity, environment etc). Anthropometric characteristics provide a better understanding of the growth process by describing changes in the body size and morphology through ages. However, all the anthropometric characteristics do not reach its peak at the same time, at the same rate or to the same extent. The variation may be evident between anthropometric characteristics, between populations, or between sexes.

The importance of age changes in the anthropometric characteristics of healthy adults helps us to understand the process of change. A large number of studies on age-related changes have been conducted on different ethnic groups in India and abroad but the majority of these studies have focused attention on the elderly population (Chiu et al. 2000; Bose and Das Chaudhuri 2003; Ghosh 2004). Very few studies have concentrated on age changes in anthropometric characteristics during adulthood (Roy and Pal 2003; Bose et al. 2006a).

India is developing countries where tribes constitute around 8.6% of the total population (Census of India 2011). In recent time, planners, researchers and administrators have drawn their attention on various tribal communities for developmental measures. Most of the tribal populations reside in rural areas of this country and they are also socially and economically underprivileged (Mittal and Srivastava 2006; Ghosh and Bharati 2006). The total number of tribal communities in West Bengal is forty (40), which constitutes 5.8% of the population in this state. Many scholars have undertaken anthropometric and nutritional assessment of different ethnic groups in West Bengal (Bose et al. 2006b; Bose et al. 2006c; Ghosh and Bharati 2006; Mittal and Srivastava 2006; Biswas 2007; Datta Banik et al. 2007; Ghosh and Malik 2007; Mondal 2007; Bisai et al. 2008; Das and Bose 2010; Das et al. 2012, Ghosh and Bose 2015).

## Objective

The present study investigated age-related trends of anthropometric characteristics and nutritional status of adult (18+ years) Mahali female residents in Bankura District. To the best of our knowledge, this is the first nutritional study among Mahali females of West Bengal.

## MATERIALS AND METHODS

Our study was conducted at four villages: Bagdiha, Rajamela, Harivanga and Gorurbasa under Chhatna and Gangajolghati blocks of Bankura district, West Bengal, India (Figure 1). These villages are located 15 km from Bankura town, which is approximately 215 km from Kolkata, the state capital of West Bengal. Prior permission and ethical approval were obtained from local community leaders as well as relevant authorities before the commencement of the study.

A total of 118 adult Mahali women aged above 18 years in those village areas were included.

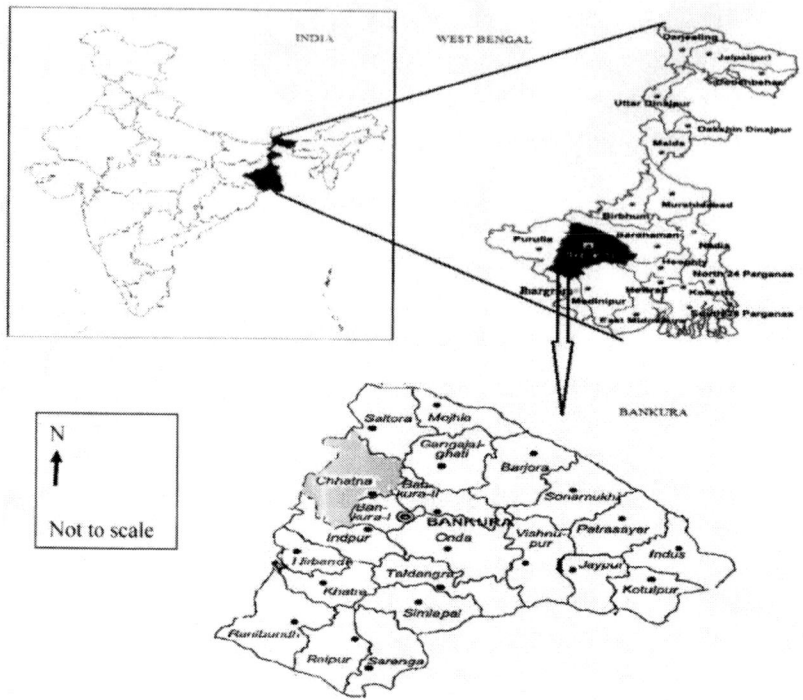

Figure 1. Location of the field area.

The socio-economic and anthropometric data were collected in pre-tested questionnaire schedule. For all study participants, the same measuring equipment was used, which were calibrated daily for standardization to reduce bias or error. All anthropometric measurements were made by two trained investigators (SB and MG) using the standard techniques of Lohman et al. (1988). Height, circumferences measurements and weight were recorded to the nearest 0.1 cm and 0.5 kg, respectively. Technical errors of measurements (TEM) were computed and were found to be within acceptable limits (Ulijaszek and Kerr 1999).

For nutritional assessment, the Body Mass Index (BMI) was computed using the following standard equation: BMI = Weight (kg) /height (m²). Nutritional status was evaluated using internationally accepted BMI guidelines (WHO, 1995). The following cut-off points were used:

Chronic Energy Deficiency (CED): BMI < 18.5;
Normal: BMI = 18.5 - 24.9
Overweight: BMI ≥ 25.0

CED was further divided into CED III, CED II, and CED I as BMI < 16.0, 16.0 - 16.9 and 17.0 -18.4 kg/m$^2$, respectively. We followed the World Health Organization's classification (1995) of the public health problem of low BMI, based on adult populations worldwide. This classification categorises prevalence according to the percentage of a population with BMI < 18.5.

Low (5-9%): warning sign, monitoring required.
Medium (10-19%): poor situation.
High (20-39%): serious situation.
Very high (≥40%): critical situation.

All statistical analyses were undertaken using the Statistical Package for Social Sciences (SPSS, version 16.0) program.One of the major limitations of our study was the small sample size.

## Area and People

Bankura district has been described as the "connecting link between the plains of Bengal on the east and Chhota Nagpur plateau on the west." The areas to the east and north-east are low-lying alluvial plains while to the west the surface gradually rises, giving way to the undulating country, interspersed with rocky hillocks. Bankura district is situated between 22° 38' and 23° 38' N latitude and 86° 36' and 87° 46' E longitude. On the north and north-east, the district is bounded by Burdwan district, from which it is separated mostly by the Damodar River. On the southeast, it is bounded by Hooghly district, on the south by Paschim Medinipur district and on the west by Purulia district. It has a total geographical area of 6,882 km². Mahali is an ethnic group inhabiting in the Chotanagpur region of

Bihar and adjoining part of Odisha and West Bengal. They are also found in Nepal and Bangladesh. According to 2011 census, a total 81,594 Mahalis are inhabitants of West Bengal of whom 49.93% are males and 50.07% are females. The sex ratio is 1002.80. Mahalis constitute 2.38% of the total population of Bankura district. Population trends indicate that Mahalis are decreasing in number. The name Mahali has been derived from the Santal word 'Mat', meaning bamboo. The Mahali language has been derived from a dialect of Santali. With their traditional occupation hierarchy, the Mahali tribes are segregated in 5 sub-groups i.e., Patar Mahali or Ghasi Mahali, Tanti Mahali, Munda Mahali, Bansphor Mahali, and Sulukhi Mahali. The Mahali tribes traditionally meet the demands of their sustenance mainly by selling items made of bamboo. The people of the tribal community are also engaged in cultivation, agricultural labour, daily labourer, collecting forest products etc.

## RESULTS

The study population of the present investigation consisted of 118 women aged 18-70 years with mean age of the participants being 33.95 ± 12.89 years. All individuals were categorized into three discreet age group categories following classification by 25th and 75th percentile, i.e., Group A: < 30 years (N = 59); Group B: 31-49 years (N = 36), and Group C: ≥ 50 years (N = 23) respectively. Table 1 presents the age group differences in mean anthropometric characteristics. There were significant age group differences in means of most of the variables and indices. Among all anthropometric variables, there existed significant age group differences in mean height ($F = 3.185$, $p < 0.05$); weight ($F = 4.44$, $p < 0.05$); sitting height ($F = 6.630$, $p < 0.05$) and medial calf ($F = 7.345$, $p < 0.05$) but not in knee height, mid-upper arm circumference and BMI ($F = 1.136$, $2.502$ and $2.178$, respectively) (Table 1). The lowest mean height, weight, sitting-height, knee-height, MUAC, medial calf and BMI were found into age group C (143.4 ± 5.47cm; 35.1 ± 5.77 kg; 71.4 ± 4.05 cm; 39.3 ± 5.59 cm; 21.1 ± 2.12 cm; 26.9 ± 2.32 cm and 17.0 ± 2.30 kg/m$^2$, respectively).

Correlation studies of age with all anthropometric indices (except knee height, MUAC and BMI) showed significant negative associations. Linear regression analyses were undertaken with age as the independent variable. Results revealed that (Table 2), age had significant impact on all variables except knee height, MUAC and BMI. A significant negative impact was observed for height (t = -2.244), weight (t = -2.633), sitting height (t = -3.545) and medial calf (t = -3.309). The amount of variation explained by age ranged from 0.8% (knee-height) to 9.0% (sitting height).

Table 3 shows the prevalence of among the participants. A total 75 individuals had CED. The distribution of CED (%) among different age groups is also presented in Table 3. The prevalence of CED was similar in all subcategories (CED I = 22.88%; CED III = 21.19% and CED II = 19.49%). There was a distinct increasing trend in the prevalence of total CED with increasing age (Group A = 5.93%, Group B = 66.67% and Group C = 78.26%).

## DISCUSSION

Anthropometric measurements have become an important tool for measuring changes in body size and body composition among populations at certain ages (Bose et al. 2003; Zverev and Chisi, 2004; Kikafunda and Lukwago, 2005; Das and Roy, 2010). These changes vary between individuals and also ethnic groups (Susanne 1980). Several international (Bose 2002) and national (Bose et al., 2003) studies have reported on the effects of age on anthropometry from the different parts of the world. However, research among tribal population of India is scanty (Sarkar and Mukhopadhyay 2008; Das and Roy 2010; Das et al. 2012). The present study demonstrated that a significant age variation existed in the anthropometric traits like weight, height, sitting height and medial calf among adult Mahali women. These results are in concordance with studies from other parts of the world on different population (Roy and Pal 2003; Sadhukan et al. 2007; Sarkar and Mukhopadhyay 2008; Das and Roy 2010; Das et al. 2012).

## Table 1. Descriptive statistics of the participants

Descriptive statistics for anthropometric parameters

| Age group in years | N | Height in cm | Weight in kg | Sitting-height in cm | Knee-height in cm | MUAC in cm | Medial-calf circumference in cm | BMI in kg/m$^2$ |
|---|---|---|---|---|---|---|---|---|
| | | Mean ± SD | Mean ± SD | Mean ± SD | Mean ± SD | Mean ± SD | Mean ± SD | Mean ± SD |
| 18-30 | 59 | 146.6±5.0 | 39.3±5.8 | 74.9±3.9 | 41.2±5.3 | 22.6±2.4 | 27.6±2.1 | 18.2±2.4 |
| 31-49 | 36 | 146.3±5.6 | 38.4±5.3 | 73.7±3.9 | 41.0±4.8 | 22.2±3.2 | 26.8±2.4 | 17.9±2.3 |
| ≥50 | 23 | 143.4±5.5 | 35.1±5.8 | 71.4±4.0 | 39.3±5.6 | 21.1±2.1 | 25.5±2.1 | 17.0±2.30 |
| Age group combined | 118 | 145.9±5.4 | 38.2±5.8 | 73.9±4.1 | 40.8±5.2 | 22.2±2.6 | 26.9±2.3 | 17.9±2.40 |
| One-Way ANOVA | | F=3.185, p<0.05 | F=4.44, p<0.05 | F=6.630, p<0.05 | F=1.163, NS | F=2.502, NS | F=7.345, p<0.05 | F=2.178, NS |

N = Number of Individuals,
SD = Standard Deviation,
MUAC = Mid Upper Arm Circumference,
BMI= Body Mass Index,
ANOVA = Analysis of Variance.

Table 2. Linear regression between age and anthropometric characteristics

| Variables | B | SeB | Beta | Adj. $R^2$ | T |
|---|---|---|---|---|---|
| Height | -0.086 | 0.038 | -0.204 | 0.033 | -2.244* |
| Weight | -0.107 | 0.041 | -0.237 | 0.048 | -2.633* |
| Sitting-height | -0.101 | 0.028 | -0.313 | 0.09 | -3.545* |
| Knee-height | -0.052 | 0.038 | -0.128 | 0.008 | -1.393 |
| MUAC | -0.033 | 0.019 | -0.136 | 0.018 | -1.781 |
| Medial calf | -0.053 | 0.016 | -0.294 | 0.078 | -3.309* |
| BMI | -0.031 | 0.017 | -0.167 | 0.02 | -1.825 |

*= Significant, $p < 0.05$.

Table 3. Age group wise prevalence of Chronic Energy of Deficiency (CED)

| Nutritional status | Age groups | | | | | | | | Total | |
|---|---|---|---|---|---|---|---|---|---|---|
| | 18-30 years | % | 31-49 years | % | >50 years | % | | | | % |
| CED-III | 11 | 18.64 | 6 | 16.67 | 8 | 34.78 | | | 25 | 21.19 |
| CED-II | 12 | 20.34 | 7 | 19.44 | 4 | 17.39 | | | 23 | 19.49 |
| CED-I | 10 | 16.95 | 11 | 30.56 | 6 | 26.09 | | | 27 | 22.88 |
| Total CED | 33 | 55.93 | 24 | 66.67 | 18 | 78.26 | | | 75 | 63.56 |
| Normal | 24 | 40.68 | 12 | 33.33 | 5 | 21.74 | | | 41 | 34.75 |
| Over | 2 | 3.39 | 0 | 0.00 | 0 | 0.00 | | | 2 | 1.69 |

## Table 4. Mean height and weight of tribal females of West Bengal: A comparison with the present study

| References | Tribe | Study area | n | Age (yrs) | Height (cm) | Weight (kg) |
|---|---|---|---|---|---|---|
| Bisai et al., 2008 | Kora Mudi | Paschim Medinipur | 123 | 34.8 | 149.3 | 40.9 |
| Biswas, 2007 | Bhumij | Paschim Medinipur | 185 | 33.8 | 148.4 | 40.5 |
| Bose et al., 2006b | Kora Mudi | Bankura | 250 | 31.7 | 147.5 | 39.5 |
| Bose et al., 2006c | Santal | Paschim Medinipur | 213 | 35.6 | 149.8 | 43.4 |
| Das and Bose, 2010 | Santal | Purulia | 317 | 37.6 | 147.5 | 39.5 |
| Datta Banik et al., 2007 | Dhimal | Darjeeling | 146 | 32.8 | 152.4 | 44.6 |
| Ghosh and Bharati, 2006 | Munda | Kolkata | 234 | 18-60 | 149.6 | 39.8 |
| Ghosh and Malik, 2007 | Santal | Bankura | 400 | 48.6 | 148.9 | 41.4 |
| Mittal and Srivastava, 2006 | Oraon | Jalpaiguri | 150 | 20-45 | 144.0 | 41.0 |
| Mondal, 2007 | Lodha | Paschim Medinipur | 199 | 34.4 | 149.2 | 42.9 |
| Ghosh et al., 2018 | Sabar | Bankura | 115 | - | 149.0 | 40.1 |
| *Present study* | *Mahali* | *Bankura* | *118* | *33.9* | *145.9* | *38.2* |

## Table 5. Mean Body Mass Index of tribal females of West Bengal: A comparison with the present study

| References | Tribe | Study Area | n | Mean BMI±SD | CED (%) | Nutritional Condition |
|---|---|---|---|---|---|---|
| Ghosh, 2007 | Bhumij | Paschim Medinipur | 185 | 18.4±2.9 | 58.9 | Critical |
| Bisai et al., 2008 | Kora Mudi | Paschim Medinipur | 123 | 18.3±2.1 | 55.3 | Critical |
| Bose et al., 2006b | Kora Mudi | Bankura | 250 | 18.3 | 56.4 | Critical |
| Bose et al., 2006c | Santal | Paschim Medinipur | 213 | 19.3±2.6 | 41.8 | Critical |
| Das and Bose, 2010 | Santal | Purulia | 317 | 18.1±2.2 | 63.4 | Critical |
| Datta Banik et al., 2007 | Dhimal | Darjeeling | 146 | 19.1±2.6 | 46.4 | Critical |
| Ghosh and Bharati, 2006 | Munda | Kolkata | 234 | 17.7±1.8 | 67.9 | Critical |
| Ghosh and Malik, 2007 | Santal | Bankura | 400 | 18.7 | 52.5 | Critical |
| Mittal and Srivastava, 2006 | Oraon | Jalpaiguri | 150 | 19.7±2.4 | 31.7 | Serious |
| Mondal, 2007 | Lodha | Paschim Medinipur | 199 | 19.3±2.6 | 40.7 | Critical |
| Ghosh et al., 2018 | Sabar | Bankura | 115 | 18.1±2.3 | 56.5 | Critical |
| *Present study* | *Mahali* | *Bankura* | *118* | *17.9±2.4* | *63.6* | *Critical* |

In the Indian context, the significant age variation in anthropometric of tribal adult women was similar to that reported among tribal populations from a different part of India (Sarkar and Mukhopadhyay 2008; Das and Roy 2010; Das et al. 2012).

The results of the present study indicated that the prevalence of undernutrition among Mahali women was notably high among all individuals. It has been suggested that undernutrition may be due to reduction of lean body mass, reduced appetite, loss of interest in food consumption and social taboo on food intake with increasing ages (Clarke et al. 1998). These are probably some of the reasons that led to under-nutrition among a large majority (78.26%) of Mahali female individuals belonging to age group 50 years and above. Furthermore, at the age groups 18 - 30 years and 31 - 49 years, Mahali females (55.93% and 66.67%, respectively) also reported nutritional stress associated with increasing age.

The comparison of mean height and weight between Mahali females and other tribal females of various districts of West Bengal state is presented in Table 3. It is clear that Mahali females of Bankura (145.9 cm) were shorter than others, except Oraons. In case of weight, the females studied by us (38.2 kg) were lighter than other tribal females of West Bengal.

The mean BMI among Mahali females were lower (17.9 kg/m$^2$) than all other tribal females except Mundas (17.7 kg/m$^2$). Similarly, the prevalence of CED was highest among Mahalis (63.6%) compared to all other tribals except Mundas (67.9%).

# CONCLUSION

Among Mahali women, age and nutritional status was significantly inversely related to anthropometric indices. This could have serious health consequences.

Furthermore, there is an urgent need for future studies to ascertain the relationship of this high rate of undernutrition among Mahali females with morbidity and mortality among this group.

## Acknowledgments

The authors thank the administrative officers and the participants for their cooperation. Financial assistance for fieldwork from the Department of Anthropology, Vidyasagar University is gratefully acknowledged under UGC SAP (DRS-I) scheme. University Grants Commission of India is also acknowledged for financial support to SP in the form of Senior Research Fellowship (Ref. No.: 590/ (NET/DEC.2013).

## Author's Contribution

SB and MG collected the data. BKK undertook data entry, analysed the data and prepared the draft manuscript. SP undertook data analyses and prepared and finalized the manuscript, KB and SP prepared and finalized the manuscript.

## Conflicts of Interest

Authors have confirmed that there is no conflict of interests.

## References

Bisai, S., Bose, K., Khatun, A., Ganguli, S., Das, P., Dikshit, S., Pradhan, S. and Mishra, T. "Nutritional stress in Kora Mudis of two districts in West Bengal. India: A comparative statement". In *Environment Pollution, Protection and Policy Issues,* edited by Saikat Kumar Basu and Sudip Datta Banik, 379-389. New Delhi: APH Publication Corporation, 2008.

Biswas, P. *Assessment of anthropometric characteristics, body composition and nutritional status of Bhumij women of Kharagpur,*

*Paschim Midnapur, West Bengal, India*. MSc dissertation, Vidyasagar University, Midnapore, West Bengal, India, 2007.

Bose, K. "Age trends in adiposity and central body fat distribution among adult white men resident in Peterborough, East Anglia, England". *Collegium Anthropologicum,* 26, no. 1 (2002): 179-186.

Bose, K., Banerjee, S., Bisai, S., Mukhopadhyay, A. and Bhadra, M. "Anthropometric profile and chronic energy deficiency among adult Santal tribals of Jhargram, West Bengal, India: Comparison with other tribal populations of Eastern India". *Ecology of Food and Nutrition,* 45, no. 3 (2006c): 159-169.

Bose, K., Bisai, S. and Chakraborty, F. "Age variations in anthropometric and body composition characteristics and underweight among male Bathudis: A tribal population of Keonjhar District, Orissa, India". *Collegium Anthropologicum,* 30, no. 4 (2006a): 771-775.

Bose, K., Das Chaudhuri, A. B. "Age variations in adiposity and body fat composition among older Bengalee Hindu women of Calcutta, India". *Anthropologischer Anzeiger,* 61, no. 3 (2003): 311-321.

Bose, K., Ganguli, S., Mamtaz, H., Mukhopadhyay, A. and Bhadra, M. "High prevalence of undernutrition among adult Kora-Mudi tribals of Bankura District, West Bengal, India". *Anthropological Science,* 114, no. 1 (2006b): 65-68.

Bose, K., Ghosh, A., Roy, S. and Gangopadhyay, S. "Blood pressure and waist circumference: an empirical study of the effects of waist circumference on blood pressure among Bengalee male jute workers of Belur, West Bengal, India". *Journal of Physiological Anthropology and Applied Human Science,* 22, no. 4 (2003): 169 - 173.

Chiu, H. C., Chang, H. Y., Mau, L. W., Lee, T. K. and Liu, H. W. "Height, weight, and body mass index of elderly persons in Taiwan". *The Journals of Gerontology Series A: Biological Sciences and Medical Sciences,* 55, no. 11 (2000): M684-M690.

Clarke, D. M., Walhqvist, M. L. and Strauss, B. J. G. "Undereating and undernutrition in old age: integrating bio-psychosocial aspects". *Age and Ageing,* 27, no. 4 (1998): 527 - 534.

Das, B. M. and Roy, S. K. "Age changes in the anthropometric and body composition characteristics of the Bishnupriya Manipuris of Cachar district, Assam". *Advances in Bioscience and Biotechnology,* 1, no. 2 (2010): 122-130.

Das, S. and Bose, K. "Body Mass Index and Chronic Energy Deficiency among Adult Santals of Purulia District, West Bengal, India". *International Journal of Human Sciences,* 7, no. 2 (2010): 488-503.

Das, S., Chowdhury, T. and Bose, K. "Age variations in anthropometric and body composition characteristics among adult Bauri females of Paschim Medinipur, West Bengal, India". *Scholarly Journal of Scientific Research and Essay Writing,* 1, no. 2 (2012): 16-24.

Datta Banik S., Bose, K., Bisai, S., Bhattacharya, M., Das, S., Jana, A. and Purkait, P. "Chronic energy deficiency among adult Dhimals of Naxalbari, West Bengal: Comparison with other tribes of Eastern India". *Food and Nutrition Bulletin,* 28, no. 3 (2007): 348-352.

Ghosh, A. "Age and sex variation in measures of body composition among the elderly Bengalee Hindus of Calcutta, India". *Collegium Anthropologicum,* 28, no. 2 (2004): 553-561.

Ghosh, M. "Nutritional status of adult Bhumij males of Kharagpur, Paschim Medinipur". In *Approaching Development, Department of Anthropology, Vidyasagar University, Midnapore, West Bengal, India,* 2007. Abstract no. 5, 22.

Ghosh, M., Bhandari, S. and Bose, K. "Anthropometric characteristics and nutritional status of adult Sabars of Bankura District, West Bengal". *Human Biology Review,* 7, no. 1 (2018): 71-83.

Ghosh, M. and Bose, K. "Assessment of Nutritional Status among male Bhumij of West Bengal, India: A comparison of body mass index and mid-upper arm circumference". *Human Biology Review,* 4, no. 2 (2015): 140-149.

Ghosh, R. and Bharati, P. "Nutritional status of adults among Munda and Pod populations in a peri-urban area of Kolkata City, India". *Asia Pacific Journal of Public Health,* 18, no. 2 (2006): 12-20.

Ghosh, S. and Malik, L. S. "Sex Differences in Body Size and Shape among Santhals of West Bengal". *Anthropologist,* 9, no. 2 (2007): 143-149.

Kikafunda, J. K. and Lukwago, F. B. "Nutritional status and functional ability of the elderly aged 60 to 90 years in the Mpigi district of central Uganda". *Nutrition,* 21, no. 1 (2005): 59-66.

Lohman, T. G., Roche, A. F. and Martorell, R. *Anthropometric Standardization Reference Manual.* Chicago: Human Kinetics Books, 1988.

Mittal, P. C. and Srivastava, S. "Diet, nutritional status and food related traditions of Oraon tribes of New Mal (West Bengal), India". *Rural and Remote Health,* 6, no. 1 (2006): 385.

Mondal, P. S. "Nutritional status of adult Lodha males of Shyamraipur, Paschim Medinipur". In *Approaching Development, Department of Anthropology, Vidyasagar University, Midnapore, West Bengal, India,* 2007. Abstract no. 6, 23.

Office of the Registrar General and Census Operation, Ministry of Home Affairs, Government of India. *Census of India.* New Delhi, India, 2011.

Roy, S. K. and Pal, B. "Anthropometric and physiological traits: Age changes among the Oraon agricultural labourer of the Jalpaiguri district, Northern West Bengal, India". *Anthropologischer Anzeiger,* 61, no. 4 (2003): 445-460.

Sadhukhan, S. K., Bose, K., Mukhopadhyay, A. and Bhadra, M. "Age variations in overweight men and women in rural areas of Hooghly District, West Bengal". *Indian Journal of Public Health,* 51, no. 1 (2007): 59 - 61.

Sarkar, S. and Mukhopadhyay, B. "Age Trends in Blood Pressure and Obesity among the Urban Bhutias of Sikkim". In *Tribes and Tribals,* special volume No. 2, *Health and Nutritional Problems of Indigenous Populations,* edited by Kaushik Bose, 59-66. New Delhi: Kamla-Raj Enterprises, 2008.

Susanne, C. "Aging, continuous changes of adulthood". In *Human Physical Growth and Maturation,* edited by Francis E. Johnston, Alex

F. Roche and Charles Susanne, 203-218. New York: Springer, Boston, MA, 1980. https://doi-org/10.1007/978-1-4684-6994-3_13.

Ulijaszek, S. J. and Kerr, D. A. "Anthropometric measurement error and the assessment of nutritional status". *British Journal of Nutrition,* 82, no. 3 (1999): 165-177.

World Health Organization. "Physical status: The use of and interpretation of anthropometry, Report of a WHO Expert Committee".*Technical Report Series,* No. 854. Geneva: World Health Organization, (1995).

Zverev, Y. and Chisi, J. "Anthropometric indices in rural Malawians aged 45-75 years". *Annals of Human Biology,* 31, no. 1 (2004): 29-37.

# INDEX

## A

addiction, ix, 3, 14, 16, 47, 57, 60
adiposity, 21, 33, 54, 55, 94
adulthood, 56, 58, 82, 96
adults, ix, 52, 54, 63, 82, 95
age, v, vii, viii, x, 2, 4, 5, 12, 13, 17, 29, 35, 39, 47, 60, 67, 68, 71, 77, 81, 82, 83, 86, 87, 88, 89, 90, 92, 94, 95, 96
age-related diseases, 71, 77
agriculture, 79
alcohol abuse, 3
alcohol consumption, viii, 2, 3, 14, 17, 19, 22, 25, 26, 31, 34, 35, 36, 37, 38, 39, 40, 41, 42, 43, 45, 46, 49, 50, 52, 53, 54, 55, 57, 58, 59, 60, 62
alcohol use, 5, 34
alcohol withdrawal, 48
alcoholic cardiomyopathy, 50
alcoholic liver disease, 4
alcoholics, ix, 2, 16, 21, 22, 29, 35, 37, 38, 39, 40, 42, 43, 44, 45
aldosterone, 36, 48
alkaline phosphatase, 44, 52
angiotensin converting enzyme, 36

anthropometric characteristics, 82, 83, 86, 89, 93
apoptosis, 33, 49
appetite, 32, 38, 41, 53, 59, 61, 92
artery, 8, 30, 36

## B

bargaining, ix, 63, 64, 65, 72, 78, 79
bargaining power, ix, 63, 64, 65, 72, 78, 79
bioavailability, 59
blood, viii, 2, 8, 20, 30, 33, 36, 44, 47, 48, 49, 50, 52, 54, 57, 94
blood pressure, 8, 20, 47, 48, 49, 55, 57, 94
blood supply, 44
blood vessels, 30, 36
BMI, viii, 2, 8, 13, 14, 16, 17, 19, 20, 21, 31, 37, 48, 84, 85, 86, 87, 88, 89, 91, 92
body composition, viii, ix, 2, 3, 21, 22, 23, 25, 27, 29, 40, 46, 51, 54, 87, 93, 94, 95
body density, 51
body fat, ix, 2, 4, 50, 94
body mass index, viii, x, 2, 31, 50, 55, 82, 84, 88, 91, 94, 95
body weight, 8, 31, 32, 33, 38, 40, 50, 59

bone, ix, 2, 4, 10, 21, 22, 43, 44, 49, 51, 52, 53, 54
bone cells, 44
bone form, 43
bone mass, 44
bone mineral content, 49

## C

calcium, 36, 43, 44, 48, 49, 52, 60
caloric intake, 33
carbon monoxide, 30
cardiovascular disease, 30, 51
central nervous system, 33, 36
children, x, 64, 69, 70, 72, 73, 74, 78, 79
cigarette smoking, 31, 39, 46, 51, 52, 59
community, viii, x, 46, 47, 50, 57, 66, 70, 78, 81, 86
composition, 47, 49, 59, 94
consumption, ix, 2, 3, 7, 14, 17, 20, 22, 25, 26, 31, 32, 34, 35, 37, 38, 39, 40, 41, 49, 50, 51, 55, 58, 60, 64, 65, 69, 92
coronary heart disease, 48, 56, 57
cortisol, 36, 38, 44, 48
cross-sectional study, viii, x, 12, 46, 81

## D

data collection, 5
development policy, 64
diastolic blood pressure, viii, 2
diastolic pressure, 36
diet, vii, viii, 1, 3, 35, 38
diseases, vii, viii, 1, 3, 15, 18, 29, 35, 46, 50, 70
distribution, 4, 50, 87, 94
dopamine, 37, 48, 61
drug addict, 60
drug addiction, 60

## E

earnings, 70, 71, 77
economic independence, 76
economic security, x, 64, 76
economic status, vii, viii, 2, 4
education, x, 6, 64, 65, 72, 76, 78, 79, 80
employment, vii, ix, 63, 64, 65, 68, 69, 71, 75, 76, 77, 78, 79, 80
employment opportunities, 76
empowerment, 64, 79, 80
endocrine disorders, 53
endothelial cells, 31
endothelial dysfunction, 33, 59
energy, x, 38, 40, 41, 47, 56, 82, 94, 95
ethanol, 39, 40, 47, 52, 53, 58, 60
ethnic groups, 82, 83, 87

## F

families, 67, 69, 70, 73, 75, 78
family budget, ix, 64, 72, 76
family budgeting, ix, 64, 72, 76
family history, viii, 2, 5, 14, 16, 34, 37
family members, 70, 76
family spending, 64, 65, 69, 71, 76
fat, ix, 2, 32, 34, 38, 40, 41, 50, 51
financial, 65, 68, 69, 93
financial support, 93
food habits, 3
food intake, 50, 57, 92
food security, 76

## G

gender differences, 60
genetic background, 38

## H

health, x, 4, 35, 44, 46, 47, 48, 52, 53, 57, 61, 64, 65, 70, 76, 82, 92
health care, 46
health condition, 35
heart attack, 30
heart disease, 3
heavy drinking, 14, 38
height, x, 8, 10, 11, 16, 19, 48, 82, 84, 86, 87, 88, 89, 90, 92
hormones, 36, 38, 44, 53
hypertension, vii, viii, 1, 40, 48, 49, 53, 56, 58, 59, 60

## I

income, 34, 64, 69, 71, 75, 76, 77, 78, 79
India, v, vii, viii, ix, x, 1, 4, 8, 29, 34, 35, 46, 47, 50, 53, 55, 56, 57, 59, 63, 64, 67, 79, 80, 81, 82, 83, 87, 92, 93, 94, 95, 96
individuals, vii, viii, x, 2, 4, 5, 12, 32, 37, 47, 58, 82, 86, 87, 92
industrialization, vii, viii, 1
insulin resistance, 33, 48, 50, 53
insulin sensitivity, 34, 39, 52, 58, 59
intra-household decision making, 65, 76, 78

## L

lean body mass, ix, 2, 92
life expectancy, 31, 56
lifestyle changes, vii, viii, 1, 3
lifestyle diseases, 3
lifetime, 7, 55, 82
light, viii, 2, 6, 7, 8, 14, 16, 21, 22, 29, 32, 35, 38, 40, 44, 45
liver cirrhosis, 54
liver damage, 51

## M

measurements, 5, 6, 10, 51, 84, 87
medical history, 4
meta-analysis, 48, 56, 57, 58
MGNREGA, v, vii, ix, 63, 64, 65, 68, 69, 70, 71, 72, 73, 74, 75, 76, 77, 78, 79
morbidity, 29, 54, 92
mortality, 4, 29, 39, 52, 92
muscle mass, ix, 2, 56, 57

## N

nicotine, 30, 32, 39, 41, 42, 49, 53
non-communicable diseases, vii, viii, 1, 3, 15, 18, 50
nutritional assessment, x, 82, 83, 84
nutritional status, v, vii, x, 81, 82, 83, 84, 89, 92, 93, 95, 96, 97

## O

obesity, vii, viii, 1, 2, 3, 4, 9, 14, 16, 20, 21, 32, 37, 38, 40, 48, 49, 50, 52, 53, 58, 59, 60, 61
old age, 77, 94
overweight, 9, 14, 16, 52, 53, 96
oxidation, 38, 41
oxidative stress, 33, 44, 59, 60

## P

parathyroid, 43, 44, 54
parathyroid hormone, 43, 44, 54
participants, x, 5, 7, 8, 82, 84, 86, 87, 88, 93
peripheral vascular disease, 44
physical activity, viii, 2, 5, 7, 31, 34, 42, 44, 53
physical inactivity, vii, viii, 1, 2, 16, 21

population, 4, 5, 7, 12, 19, 39, 50, 51, 53, 54, 55, 83, 85, 86, 87, 94
potential benefits, 5
poverty, 64, 67, 69, 75, 78, 80
poverty line, 67, 69, 75, 78
protein synthesis, 42, 60
public health, 85

## Q

questionnaire, viii, 2, 5, 7, 84

## R

recommendations, iv
regression, 74, 87, 89
regression equation, 74
response, 54, 60, 70, 74
risk, vii, viii, ix, 2, 3, 5, 12, 14, 15, 16, 18, 19, 20, 30, 33, 34, 35, 37, 38, 39, 40, 46, 47, 48, 49, 51, 54, 55, 56, 57, 58, 59, 61
risk assessment, 55
risk factors, vii, viii, ix, 2, 3, 5, 12, 14, 15, 16, 18, 19, 20, 34, 36, 46, 47, 55, 56, 58
rural areas, vii, ix, 63, 76, 77, 78, 83, 96
rural people, 35, 76
rural population, 59
rural poverty, vii, ix, 63, 78
rural women, 64, 76, 77, 78, 79

## S

savings, 69, 71, 72, 77
savings account, 72
school, x, 6, 64, 65, 69, 70, 73, 74, 75, 78
school dropout, x, 64, 65, 72, 74, 75, 78
skeletal muscle, 42
smokeless tobacco, viii, 2, 3, 15, 18, 20, 58
smoking, viii, 2, 3, 4, 12, 13, 14, 15, 16, 19, 20, 21, 23, 24, 29, 30, 31, 32, 33, 34, 35, 37, 39, 40, 41, 42, 43, 44, 45, 46, 47, 48, 49, 50, 51, 52, 53, 54, 56, 57, 58, 59, 60, 61
smoking cessation, 21, 32, 34, 44, 53, 54, 56, 57, 59
soamtotype, 3
social life, 76
social security, 64
society, vii, viii, 1, 3, 65, 76
spending, 64, 65, 69, 70, 71, 76, 77
surveillance, vii, viii, 2, 46, 61

## T

tobacco, vii, viii, 1, 2, 3, 4, 5, 7, 15, 18, 19, 20, 29, 30, 34, 39, 41, 44, 46, 49, 52, 58, 60, 61
tobacco smoke, 29, 30, 60
tobacco smoking, 19
toxic effect, 43, 44
treatment, 8, 61, 70, 76
type 2 diabetes, 48, 50, 53, 54, 56

## U

undernutrition, 92, 94
urbanization, vii, viii, 1

## V

variables, viii, x, 2, 5, 12, 14, 35, 75, 82, 86, 87
vasoconstriction, 30, 54
vitamin D, 43, 49, 55
vitamin E, 52

## W

wages, 64, 70, 72, 77, 78
wastage problem, 64, 79
weight gain, 32, 34, 49, 54, 59
weight loss, 40
withdrawal, 33, 78
withdrawal symptoms, 33
work activity, 82
workers, 64, 65, 66, 67, 68, 69, 70, 71, 72, 73, 75, 77, 78, 80, 94
worldwide, 29, 34, 85